Sports Medicine Essentials

Sports Medicine Essentials

Tobias Fry

SYRAWOOD
PUBLISHING HOUSE
New York

Published by Syrawood Publishing House,
750 Third Avenue, 9th Floor,
New York, NY 10017, USA
www.syrawoodpublishinghouse.com

Sports Medicine Essentials
Tobias Fry

International Standard Book Number: 978-1-64740-255-6 (Hardback)

Cataloging-in-Publication Data

Sports medicine essentials / Tobias Fry.
p. cm.
Includes bibliographical references and index.
ISBN 978-1-64740-255-6
1. Sports medicine. 2. Medicine. 3. Sports sciences. I. Fry, Tobias.
RC1210 .S66 2022
617.102 7--dc23

TABLE OF CONTENTS

Preface VII

Chapter 1 Introduction 1

- Sports Physiotherapy 8
- Sports Chiropractic 12
- Sport Psychology 13
- Conconi Test 16
- Diving Medicine 17
- Orthopedic Sports Medicine 28

Chapter 2 General Sports Injuries and their Treatment 36

- Ankle Injury 36
- Groin Strain 44
- Shin Pain 48
- Hamstring Injuries 51
- Knee Injury 65
- Achilles Tendon Rupture 73
- Athletic Heart Syndrome 75
- Patellar Tendinitis 76
- Female Athlete Triad 77
- Relative Energy Deficiency in Sport 81

Chapter 3 Sport-Specific Injuries and their Treatment 87

- Basketball Injuries 87
- Baseball Injuries 91
- Football Injuries 96
- Running Injuries 98
- Swimming Injuries 108
- Racquet Injuries 110
- Climbing Injuries 112

Chapter 4 **Sports Nutrition** **118**

- Nutrition for Sports Persons 118
- Fluid Balance 122
- Sports Supplements 129
- Glutamine 131
- Creatine 142
- Protein 146
- Sports Drink 153
- Types of Sports Drinks 157

Chapter 5 **Physical Therapy and Rehabilitation** **161**

- Physical Therapy 161
- Rehabilitation in Sport 164
- Therapeutic Exercise 174
- Principles of Exercise and Sport Training 176
- Exercises to Recover from a Sports Hernia 178
- Core Exercises for Athletes to Build Strength and Fight Back Pain 179

Chapter 6 **Prevention of Sports Injuries** **198**

- Baseball Injury Prevention 206
- Injury Prevention in Football 210
- Soccer Injury Prevention 213
- Prevention of Climbing Injuries 216

Permissions

Index

PREFACE

It is with great pleasure that I present this book. It has been carefully written after numerous discussions with my peers and other practitioners of the field. I would like to take this opportunity to thank my family and friends who have been extremely supporting at every step in my life.

The branch of medicine that focuses on the prevention and treatment of sports related emergencies and injuries is known as sports medicine. It also deals with physical fitness. Various injuries related to ligaments, muscles, tendons and bones are treated in sports medicine. A few of such injuries are ankle sprains, concussions, cartilage injuries and fractures. It also deals with serious illnesses, such as diabetes and asthma, which may affect the physical performance of a person. There are various specializations within this field such as orthopedic surgery, sports physical therapy, physical medicine and rehabilitation. This book is a compilation of chapters that discuss the most vital concepts and emerging trends in the field of sports medicine. It will provide comprehensive insights into this field. This book is an essential guide for both academicians and those who wish to pursue this discipline further.

The chapters below are organized to facilitate a comprehensive understanding of the subject:

Chapter - Introduction

Sports medicine is a branch of medicine that is concerned with the prevention and treatment of injuries related to sports and exercise. It includes sports physiotherapy, diving medicine, sports chiropractic, sport psychology, orthopaedic sports medicine, etc. This is an introductory chapter which will introduce briefly all the significant aspects of these branches of sports medicine.

Chapter - General Sports Injuries and their Treatment

Injuries that occur during athletic activities, sports or exercise are called sports injuries. Ankle injury, knee injury, shin pain, patellar tendinitis, groin strain, Achilles tendon rupture, athletic heart syndrome, hamstring injuries and female athlete triad are some of the common sports injuries. This chapter has been carefully written to provide an easy understanding of these types of sports injuries and their treatment.

Chapter - Sport-Specific Injuries and their Treatment

There are some injuries that are specific to particular sports such as ankle injuries in basketball, and sprains, fractures and concussions in baseball. This chapter has been carefully written to provide an easy understanding of different sports-specific injuries such as injuries related to football, swimming and racquet sports.

Chapter - Sports Nutrition

The study and practice of implementing appropriate diet and nutrition to improve the athletic performance of a person is known as sports nutrition. It studies the type and quantity of fluids and food taken by an athlete. The topics elaborated in this chapter will help in gaining a better perspective about sports nutrition as well as the different types of sports drinks which fall under it.

Chapter - Physical Therapy and Rehabilitation

Physical therapy is a type of physical rehabilitation which uses evidence-based kinesiology, exercise prescription, joint mobilization, electrotherapy and health education to treat the conditions such as soft tissue injuries, arthritis, etc. Rehabilitation seeks to restore functional ability to those with physical impairments or disabilities. The chapter closely examines the key concepts of physical therapy and rehabilitation to provide an extensive understanding of the subject.

Chapter - Prevention of Sports Injuries

Sports injury preventions are broadly classified into three categories: primary, secondary and tertiary prevention. Primary prevention involves the avoidance of injury, secondary prevention includes the early diagnosis and treatment of an injury, and tertiary prevention primarily focuses on the rehabilitation to reduce and correct an existing disability. This chapter discusses in detail the methods used to prevent injuries in various sports such as soccer and baseball.

Tobias Fry

Introduction

CHAPTER 1

Sports medicine is a branch of medicine that is concerned with the prevention and treatment of injuries related to sports and exercise. It includes sports physiotherapy, diving medicine, sports chiropractic, sport psychology, orthopaedic sports medicine, etc. This is an introductory chapter which will introduce briefly all the significant aspects of these branches of sports medicine.

Sports medicine is the medical and paramedical supervision, of athletes in training and in competition, with the goal of prevention and treatment of their injuries. Sports medicine entails the application of scientific research and practice to the optimization of health and athletic performance.

Since the revival of the Olympic Games in 1896, increased participation in sport and training for sports have resulted in the need to not only prevent and treat sports injury but also advance the scientific knowledge of the limits of human exercise performance and the causes of fatigue. Moreover, with increased training levels and specialization across the spectrum of recreational sports and with opportunities for sport participants to become professionals, there has been a parallel increase in the careers to support the care and training of athletes and physically active individuals.

Sports Medicine Specialties

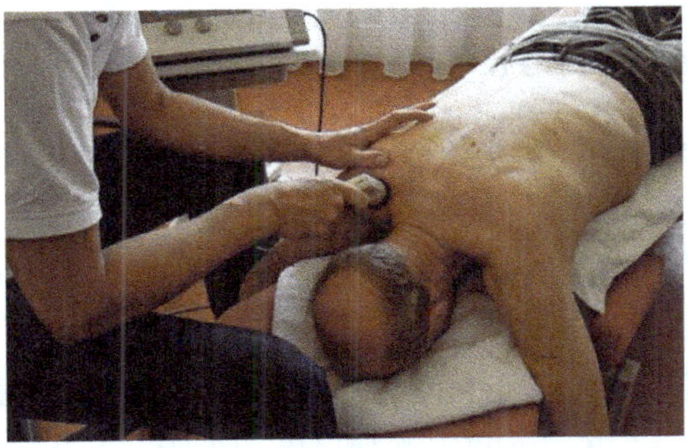

Sports medicine; physiotherapy: A physiotherapist treating the shoulder of a senior patient.

Sports medicine is an umbrella term representing a broad array of specialties that bridge the academic disciplines of medicine and physical education as well as the basic sciences (e.g., physiology, chemistry, and physics). Within clinical medicine, physicians in primary care or pediatrics may become team physicians for competitive teams at all levels (interscholastic, intercollegiate, professional, and amateur sports). Other members of a sports medicine team typically include an orthopedic surgeon, a certified athletic trainer, a physical therapist or kinesiotherapist, and a strength-and-conditioning specialist. Other professionals, such as those in the areas of sports nutrition, sports psychology, sports physiology, podiatry, sports vision, sports dentistry, and chiropractic, are valuable consultants.

Although sports medicine is more commonly thought to be related specifically to orthopedic medicine, with respect to the treatment and prevention of injuries occurring in a sport, other medical specialties in cardiology, psychiatry, gynecology, and ophthalmology can also play an important role in comprehensive sports medicine. For example, cardiac rehabilitation is an important area in sports medicine that employs not only doctors but also allied health professionals, such as registered clinical exercise physiologists and nurses. These individuals help patients recover and improve their functional capacity following cardiovascular events such as heart attack or cardiac surgery.

A sports medicine team physician can be called upon to treat a wide variety of sports-related injuries or illnesses. One example is an overuse type of injury, such as a stress fracture in the foot or lower leg. An injury such as this can be caused by any of a variety of problems, including muscle imbalance, muscular weakness arising from a lack of proper strength training, improper footwear or abnormal gait, inadequate mineral or other nutrient intake that upsets the caloric balance necessary for training, hormonal deficiency, and overload of exercise training volume, frequency, and intensity. Thus, to effectively treat an overuse injury, a team physician needs expertise and knowledge in a wide range of sports medicine issues.

Sports Medicine and Health

The use of exercise and sport as a therapy to prevent chronic disease is well established. The wide range of health benefits of exercise stem from the several key elements that comprise physical fitness: cardiorespiratory endurance, muscular strength, muscular endurance, flexibility, agility, and body composition.

The relationship between regular physical activity and health has been well established worldwide. Governments of numerous countries have published guidelines that describe the amount of physical activity needed for health, although these guidelines may vary slightly.

In 2008 the U.S. government released Physical Activity Guidelines for Americans, the country's first published set of guidelines on the "dose," or amount, of physical activity needed to maintain health for individuals aged six and older. This document was based on a rigorous review by an expert panel of the scientific literature available on exercise and health. The panel found strong evidence indicating that 150 minutes of moderate to vigorous exercise per week for adults helped prevent a wide range of diseases, including cardiovascular disease, stroke, diabetes, hypertension (high blood pressure), certain types of cancer, and depression. This amount of exercise for adults was also associated with a reduced risk of early death, of falls, and of weight gain. There was also moderate evidence indicating that this level of physical activity aids in the prevention of hip fracture, osteoporosis, lung cancer, and endometrial cancer; facilitates weight maintenance after weight loss; and improves sleep quality.

The 2008 U.S. report also indicated that for individuals aged 6 to 17 the baseline dose of exercise needed to obtain health benefits was 60 minutes or more of physical activity every day (physical activity was defined as aerobic or endurance exercise of moderate or vigorous intensity). The greatest health benefits were associated with vigorous activity at least three days per week. Muscle-strengthening and bone-strengthening activities performed at least three days per week for children and at least two days per week for adults were also found to improve health.

In Canada, youths are encouraged to obtain even more minutes of daily activity (60 moderate and 30 vigorous minutes). In general, similar guidelines have been established for all individuals, and they are not considered to be optimal training doses for various sports and athletes. Training for competitive sports generally requires additional sports medicine expertise.

Exercise in therapeutic doses is powerful in preventive medicine. Therefore, in the broadest of terms, sports medicine is applicable to any individual who includes movement as a part of his or her daily life as well as to those who compete on teams or in individual sports—from youth to masters-level events.

There is no universally accepted definition of sports and exercise medicine (SEM). The nature of the discipline has changed over time and continues to do so as SEM begins to clarify its scope more clearly and delineates itself from the traditional medical specialties. This lack of a universal concept of SEM raises a number of dangers for the future development of the specialty that is starting to become apparent. By its very nature, the process of recognition of SEM as a new medical specialty means that the scope of the field has to be defined in government regulations.

This formalised definition then has the potential to be hijacked by competing priorities between clinical SEM practitioners who have evolved the specialty over time and health department civil servants who are looking for ways and means to obviate the growing public health burden associated with inactivity. Although the two views share common ground, the underpinning philosophy is fundamentally different and this subtle burocratic re-focussing directly influences training and how the field of SEM evolves in the future.

Current day clinicians need to be clear that this process of SEM governance serves their view of the specialty correctly. Governing councils and faculties should reflect clinical SEM rather than the view of SEM that other specialties and civil servants think should be in place. It is a very real danger that we could finish up training public health physicians with little in the way of SEM competency rather than what we need, which is SEM specialists with competency in public health medicine.

Traditional vs. New Models of SEM

Emerging and novel concepts, a new generation of trainees untrammeled by history and the overwhelming desire for SEM to take its place amongst the panoply of mainstream specialties all help drive the evolution of the specialty in new directions. The fact that this emerging discipline is not organ, system or disease specific both allows these possibilities and creates some of the very real dangers that threaten the existence of the specialty.

The traditional role of SEM began as a form of individual athlete and team care particularly at the elite level. Not surprisingly the emergence of the discipline has been closely linked to the Olympic movement and more recently the proliferation of professional sport and their needs for high quality medical coverage. Throughout the world, a generation of SEM physicians has developed from either a primary care or orthopaedic background and the specialty itself has then developed into an independent consultant level of expertise and broadened to encompass the management of a range of medical problems associated with exercise.

This role of the SEM specialist utilising their underpinning musculoskeletal medicine skills treating complex or chronic medical conditions remains a promising development but is likely to have a limited take up unless the specialty is recognised more widely, numbers of consultant level SEM specialists increase substantially and existing cognate disciplines buy into this model of care.

The broader public health engagement of SEM practitioners to promote health and prevent disease at a population level remains difficult to judge at this time. The UK Department of Health recognised this role as one of the key reasons for the recognition of SEM as a specialty. Given the relatively small numbers of SEM physicians, the limited training of SEM practitioners in public health medicine (when compared to existing pubic health practitioners) coupled with the lack of SEM specific representation at a policy level, it remains to be seen whether this promise will be ultimately fulfilled.

This then raises a disturbing issue that in countries where the training is orientated to public health concepts (eg UK) the risk is that this model of training will not adequately equip SEM practitioners for a future leadership role in public health and their core musculoskeletal sports medicine skills will be limited due to the needs of their curriculum to cover such public health and other skills. Conversely countries with an exercise and injury focus (eg Australia/New Zealand) may have better clinical competency to deal with the medical problems of exercise as well as utilising exercise in the treatment of complex medical problems, but would be relatively less equipped to deal with the public health aspects of SEM.

It is a brave experiment by the health burocrats in different countries where the core competency of individual SEM practitioners will reflect these disparate views of just what the scope of SEM entails. With the various models of SEM training that exist in different countries, there is a brief window for harmonisation of skills and training that will rapidly pass. The risk is that SEM practitioners will have little in the way of "transportable" skills given the widely differing models of practice in different countries.

Who Actually does SEM?

SEM is practised in a variety of settings. The vast majority of sports injuries are currently managed by primary care practitioners and this is unlikely to substantially change in the foreseeable future given the current low numbers of SEM consultants and the relatively small numbers of specialists that can be trained annually.

Clearly there is an argument to be made for the health system or the existing SEM colleges and faculties to strengthen this situation either by up-skilling general practitioners and/or advocating for the development of a two-tiered system of care with a network of specialists supporting general practitioners for the management of complex and difficult cases.

The role and scope of specialist SEM can be seen conceptually on three levels within the continuum of health or wellness. The areas in which SEM specialists cover includes:

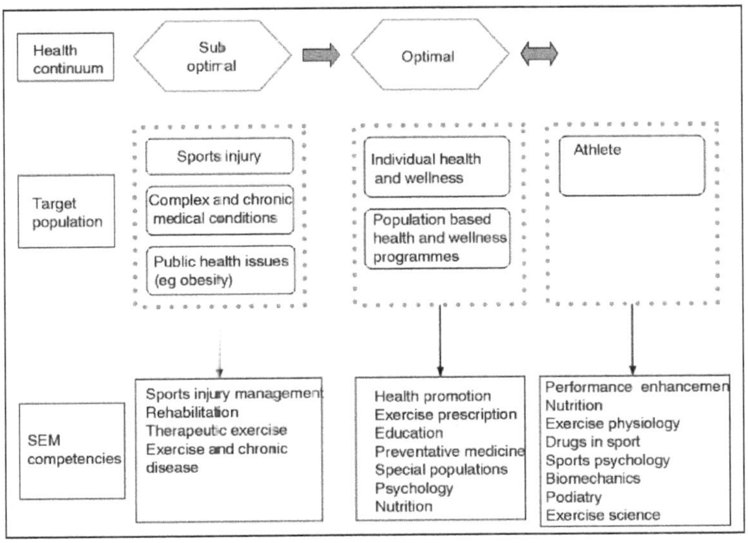

SEM health and performance continuum.

- Suboptimal health—The problems of injury related to exercise or where exercise is part of the management of medical problems either at an individual or population level.
- Optimal health—The use of exercise to maximise wellness at either individual level (exercise prescription) or at a population level (public health).
- Supra-optimal health—The use of SEM skills to enhance performance in an athletic population.

SEM by not being confined to a body system or organ exists as an area that has a range of knowledge and skills that are not unique to the discipline. Overlapping disciplines include the principal specialty areas related to musculoskeletal medicine (eg orthopedic surgery, rheumatology, rehabilitation medicine, emergency medicine, occupational medicine), primary care, public health medicine as well as a range of other specialties involved in specific problems (eg cardiology and neurology).

In some cases, cognate disciplines such as rheumatology and rehabilitation, recognise that their practitioners require skills and training in both musculoskeletal and sports medicine; however, existing specialists have largely not taken up the challenge of developing this area and few have established sub-specialty practices in SEM.

Although SEM is a distinct area of medicine, with such overlap being present and the shared clinical focus within a number of specialties, there is the potential for mutually beneficial relationships to develop with the possibility of shared training and education opportunities. Existing specialties having much to learn from SEM and vice versa.

Unified Definition of SEM

The International Federation of Sports Medicine (FIMS) has defined SEM as:

> "embodying theoretical and practical medicine which examines the influence of exercise, training and sports, as well as the lack of exercise, on healthy and unhealthy people of all ages to produce results that are conducive to prevention, therapy and rehabilitation as well as beneficial for the athlete himself".

Similarly the Royal College of Physicians (UK) uses the following definition:

> "SEM is the discipline that addresses medical conditions and injuries that occur in those who wish to participate in sport or to exercise in other ways. It also covers the role of physical activity in the treatment and prevention of illness".

The Medical Council of New Zealand has listed a burocratic definition of SEM for the purposes of vocational registration and states that:

> "The medical care of the exercising individual, including the assessment and management of patients with musculoskeletal injuries and medical problems arising from sporting activity. Sports physicians possess expertise in general medicine, orthopedics and rehabilitation plus allied sports sciences including nutrition, biomechanics, exercise physiology and sports psychology".

In Australia, the Australasian College of Sports Physicians reflect the traditional vies; however, they have broadened the scope of SEM by defining it as:

> "a wide ranging discipline incorporating aspects of disease and injury prevention, the management of the medical problems of exercising individuals, the management of soft tissue injuries sustained with exercise and the prescription

> of exercise for both improving physical fitness and treating disease. It also looks at the discrete exercise needs of certain population groups such as the elderly, those with disabilities and children. It provides expertise in the medical needs of sporting individuals, sporting teams and sporting events. It covers aspects of the medical care of individuals exercising in extreme environments and deals with pharmacological and ethical issues involved in drugs and doping in sport. Research in SEM is particularly concerned with injury prevention, enhancing physical function, understanding and improving impairment and enhancing the rehabilitation of injuries".

By contrast, the UK Intercollegiate Board of Sport and Exercise Medicine has used the following definition in its submission to the UK Dept of Health in its application for SEM specialty recognition and reflects more of a public health element than the traditional views:

"SEM is a discipline that draws upon basic and applied biomedical and clinical sciences for the furtherance of knowledge and ensuring best practice in the diagnosis and management of SEM clinical problems. The discipline is relevant to the whole population and seeks to promote health, to prevent disease or injury, to apply optimal treatment and rehabilitation and to measure outcomes".

By taking elements of the definitions above, the conceptual understanding of SEM and examining the evidence for the specific roles of SEM physicians, a new definition is proposed below.

SEM can be defined as a broad ranging discipline incorporating the:

- Management of the medical problems of exercising individuals at all ages and all levels of participation.
- The pathophysiology, biomechanics and optimisation of human performance.
- The use of exercise as a therapeutic modality in the treatment and prevention of disease.
- The promotion of health and the prevention of disease or injury at a population level.

The first two of these areas are the "traditional" view of SEM and would be universally agreed upon, point 3 represents the short to medium term evolution but still requires engagement by traditional medical specialties in order to become a reality, and point 4 is a long-term goal whilst having enormous potential remains unproven at the present time.

Priorities in the Scope of SEM Reflect Training

Could one therefore make an argument that training should reflect these priorities proposed in this new definition with most of the focus on the management of the medical problems of exercising individuals and the optimisation of human performance rather than public health?

The limited development of SEM in particular countries makes this problematic.

In the UK, there are virtually no hospital posts or even true sports medicine clinics where there are experienced and competent SEM practitioners with an ample sports injury patient load where supervised training could be done. There are, however, numerous practitioners who practice a diverse range of "wellness" and occupational medicine where some aspects of training could occur; however, this could not deliver the necessary competency training. In Australia, the US, Canada, New Zealand and various countries in Europe, the development of specialist SEM clinics through the private sector as well as the government funded institutes of sport means that this training limitation is less problematic.

Is the priority public health? Although attractive to health departments and with a clear need given the national health priorities related to the medical effects of inactivity, it is easy to see why funding bodies responsible for training will try to influence the core curriculum to push this particular focus. The problem, however, is that without substantive funding quarantined for SEM, it is unlikely that this will become a reality in the foreseeable future. In the UK, a handful of training places are being negotiated with the postgraduate deans who themselves are under increasing budgetary pressures within the health system. The government seems to recognise the need (at least in various published reports) but seems unwilling to fund this development.

What are the Risks to SEM?

One of the risks of the specialty of SEM is that it will be hijacked by civil servants who are pushing a public health agenda but without adequate funding to make this concept a reality. In addition, that governance of SEM increasingly is seen to be dominated by those in traditional specialties (eg orthopedic surgery) who have little conceptual understanding of the underlying nature of SEM itself. The end result is a cohort of SEM physicians who lack the necessary SEM competencies to have a globally transportable skill set and may well not have sufficient public health expertise to satisfy the agenda of the bureaucrats. SEM physicians need to be very clear as to what the future holds.

SPORTS PHYSIOTHERAPY

Sports Physiotherapy is an evidence-based discipline that offers evaluation, prevention and rehabilitation/treatment of sports injuries, and it also focuses on performance enhancement.

Whether you are a competitive athlete, exercise recreationally or want to kick start an active healthy lifestyle, our team of physiotherapists will see to your needs. An experienced team of Sports Physiotherapists and physiotherapist assistants stay up-to date on the latest evidence based therapy practices and techniques to speed up patient's recovery and help achieve their functional goals.

Sports physiotherapy techniques involve hands on, individualized, manual therapy, electrotherapy modalities, rehabilitation exercises and education. Rehabilitation exercises are an important tool for injury management, and comprise of targeted stretches, strengthening, agility, coordination, and balance exercises. Clinical pilates and proprioceptive neuromuscular facilitation techniques are also amongst the repertoire of therapeutic exercises utilised by our therapists.

Sports physiotherapy services include:

- Injury management and rehabilitation.
- Post – surgical management and rehabilitation.
- Injury prevention/education programs.
- Biomechanical analysis to correct posture, gait and sport specific technique.
- Individually tailored exercise therapy to improve flexibility, strength and coordination.
- Clinical pilates for injury management/prevention.

Benefits from Sports Physiotherapy

Value of Sport Physiotherapy

The physiotherapy profession has several areas of expertise to meet the health and mobility needs of Canadians. One specialized area of practice is Sports Physiotherapy.

Sport Physiotherapy

Sport Physiotherapy assists active Canadians of all ages and levels with injuries sustained in sport, or with illness, imbalances, and barriers that prevent maximal participation and performance in sport. In Canada, Physiotherapists who practice Sport Physiotherapy, are members of Sport Physiotherapy Canada, a Division within the Canadian Physiotherapy Association.

Practices Sport Physiotherapy

Upon graduating from an accredited University Physiotherapy program, physiotherapists can focus their time and advanced training working with athletes. Sport

Physiotherapy Canada has a credentialing system that allows members to progress their knowledge and skills through mentoring, courses, and written and practical examinations.

Specialized skills do physiotherapists have who work in sport physiotherapy:

- 'On-field' emergency care and sideline injury management.
- Organization of medical and paramedical event coverage.
- Athletic taping.
- Sports massage.
- Functional testing for return to sport decision making.
- Protective equipment analysis, fit and maintenance.
- Protective bracing selection.
- Knowledge of exercise physiology and strength and conditioning for exercise program development and modification.
- Clinical management of acute and chronic sport injuries.
- Pre-season screening for detecting medical and injury risk and establishing baselines.
- Development of programs for injury prevention.
- Concussion detection and management.

Benefits from Sport Physiotherapy

The value of Sport Physiotherapy can be determined by considering who would benefit from these specialized and advanced skills:

- General public can benefit from sport physiotherapy through expert management of acute and chronic injuries, assist with returning to training and provide advise on how to prevent Physiotherapy is a primary care profession which means that a referral is not required. This allows for timely health care access, early intervention and injury management, and prevention of secondary issues form being inactive.
- Young growing athletes and teams can benefit from education on preventing imbalances related to the developing musculoskeletal system such as inflexibility, altered coordination and movement Injury prevention education also

includes, why and how to complete proper warm-ups, cool-downs, stretching and other recovery tools. Understanding injuries and reducing fear is also important to ensure young Canadians continue with activity or sport. A special topic would also include education around Concussions in sport.

- High performance athletes benefit from almost daily interactions with sport physiotherapy as part of their collaborative sports medicine Pre-season screening and regular in-season check-ins can detect risks for injuries and provide guidance in areas requiring improved performance. With application of recovery methods, proper progression and application of exercise physiology, Sport Physiotherapy can help these athletes push their boundaries and achieve high levels of success.

- Coaches utilize the expertise of the field of sport physiotherapy in developing injury prevention programs and yearlong training schedules to get peak performance from their Communication regarding field of play injury assessment, clinical injury management and return to training modifications and planning are also essential.

- Schools and sport organizations value the input of Sport Physiotherapy to develop injury prevention and management protocols, concussion policies, injury tracking, as well as organizing and providing sports event first aid.

- Older active Canadians can be taught how to continue beloved activities despite symptoms of past injury and illnesses such as arthritis, diabetes, osteoporosis.

- Those injured at work or from motor vehicle collisions can benefit from Sport Physiotherapy's approach to return to play by applying them to return to work and daily activities through exercise-based progressions and activity Concussions sustained here can also receive the most up to date, research-based care.

- Physiotherapists wanting to provide the best care for the active Canadian population or strive for the ability to attend sports events such as the Olympics, can learn more by becoming involved with Sport Physiotherapy Canada.

- Other health care providers and fitness professionals including Family Physicians, emergency centres, Orthopedic Surgeons, Massage Therapists, Chiropractors, Osteopaths, Registered Dietitians, Personal and Team Trainers, and more, work closely with those in the field of Sport Physiotherapy to provide a collaborative environment for their active.

Physiotherapists can be found in a variety of settings including hospitals, schools, community health centres, nursing homes, fitness centres and more, but most physiotherapists involved with providing sport physiotherapy work in private practice physiotherapy clinics throughout Canada. They often work with other health care practitioners providing a multi-disciplinary approach to care.

SPORTS CHIROPRACTIC

Sports chiropractic (or chiropractic sports medicine) is a relatively new subspecialty in the field of chiropractic healing. As chiropractic care becomes more mainstream, more practitioners are starting to specialize in a variety of healing methods. Sports chiropractors specialize in the care of musculoskeletal injuries, including prevention. This branch of chiropractic expertise is an excellent resource for athletes. Whether you need a little advice on performance issues or treatment for a sport-related injury, any type of athlete will find that a sports chiropractor is an important part of keeping their body in peak condition.

Chiropractic care has been around for thousands of years, but it wasn't until 1980 that the first chiropractor was added to the United States Olympic medical team. Since then, spinal adjustments have become an important part of many sports medical teams. Athletes from every walk of life are starting to realize the long-term benefits of chiropractic care.

Sports chiropractors take a multidisciplinary approach to treat their patients. They also have an extensive knowledge of sports and sports-related injuries. This means that they're uniquely qualified to diagnose and treat an athlete's body without the use of drugs or invasive surgical procedures. Because chiropractic medicine is defined by its "hands on" approach to healing and the belief in caring for the entire body, it's becoming an increasingly popular way to stay in the game without relying on drugs or surgeries.

Sports chiropractic is a highly specialized field that typically focuses on professional or aspiring athletes. If you don't spend a good portion of your life participating in a sport, you probably don't require that level of specialized care. Your local chiropractic team is trained in the same type of spinal manipulation and pain relief techniques as a sports chiropractor, and can perform the same techniques as a specialist. They're also able to offer a more general approach to your overall health.

Every chiropractor treats injuries with the same basic techniques. They use spinal manipulation to align your spine and traction tables to relieve pressure in the discs in your back. A good chiropractor will also be eager to educate you on the proper way to move your body to avoid injury. Chiropractors are strong believers in holistic care. This means that they're concerned with the health of your whole body and can be an excellent resource for the sports-minded individual.

Anyone who plays sports regularly can benefit from chiropractic care. Your chiropractor can help you with aches and pains that come along with an exercise regimen, as well as helping you to stay fit and healthy. If exercise pains are slowing your workout down, get going to your chiropractor for an adjustment. They'll have you back at the gym in no time at all.

SPORT PSYCHOLOGY

Sport psychology is a proficiency that uses psychological knowledge and skills to address optimal performance and well-being of athletes, developmental and social aspects of sports participation, and systemic issues associated with sports settings and organizations. APA recognizes sport psychology as a proficiency acquired after a doctoral degree in one of the primary areas of psychology and licensure as a psychologist. This proficiency does not include those who have earned a doctoral degree in sport psychology but are not licensed psychologists.

Sport Psychology interventions are designed to assist athletes and other sports participants (e.g., coaches, administrators, parents) from a wide array of settings, levels of competition and ages, ranging from recreational youth participants to professional and Olympic athletes to master's level performers.

Skills and Procedures

Many strategies and procedures are used to address problems faced by athletes and other sports participants. Some of the principal areas include:

- Cognitive and behavioral skills training for performance enhancement: Goal setting; imagery and performance planning; concentration and attention control strategies; development of self-confidence, self-esteem and competence in sports; cognitive-behavioral self-regulation techniques; emotion management, sportsmanship and leadership skills.
- Counseling and clinical interventions: Athletic motivation; eating disorders and weight management; substance abuse; grief, depression, loss and suicide; over-training and burnout; sexual identity issues; aggression and violence; athletic injury and rehabilitation; career transitions and identity crises.
- Consultation and training: Team building; sports organization consultation; systems interventions with parents and families involved in youth sports participation; education of coaches regarding motivation, interpersonal and leadership skills and talent development; education of coaches and administrators regarding early identification and prevention of psychological difficulties.

Let's take a look at the field of sport psychology and discover how it can help you as an athlete, parent of an athlete, or as a coach. Here are ten areas that sport psychology studies, and how it applies this knowledge to sport learning and performance:

- Sport Psychology helps you understand yourself as an athlete: You need to have mental strategies for learning, practice and performance factors. Sport psychology gives you the methods and approaches to become aware of what you need so you and your coach can craft custom interventions.

- Sport Psychology helps you work better with your parents: Your parents should be part of your success team, at least at some level. It does not necessarily mean they should coach you, but it would be nice to have a solid relationship with them, and excellent communication skills so they can assist you in your career.

- Sport Psychology helps you work better with your coaches: Your coach is perhaps the most important person on your team. You need a great working relationship with this person. Sport psychology can help you create this relationship, and nurture it.

- Sport Psychology helps you navigate your sport career: There are many blind alleys, pitfalls and false paths in a sport career. Sport psychology helps you create a vision for success, and goals and objectives, so you can execute that master plan.

- Sport Psychology helps you prepare your mind: It is critical that you know how to prepare mentally and emotionally for lessons, practices and performances. Sport psychology helps you devise a customized mental readiness process that helps you transition from your normal work, school or social worlds into the special world of competition.

- Sport Psychology helps you concentrate so you can enter the zone: Attentional control is psychologist-speak for concentration or focus. Sport psychology helps you create strong control over where and how you place your attention so you can concentrate on the proper attentional cues, and you are able to block out unwanted, distracting cues.

- Sport Psychology helps you bounce back from set-backs: It is critical that you become resilient to the inevitable problems and set-backs that competitive sport brings. You need solid mental toughness that helps you refocus, reset and re-energize for what is to come.

- Sport Psychology helps you increase motivation and drive: Successful athletes who have long careers fuel them with exciting goals, a vision for the legacy they want to leave, and dreams of how they want to play. Sport psychology helps you craft engaging goals that create positive energy within you, so you have huge amounts of drive and determination to achieve your potential.

- Sport Psychology helps you handle stress and pressure: One of the major ways sport psychology helps you is through stress reduction in learning and performance. While some stress is inevitable and natural, levels of stress that are excessive damage performance. Sport psychology helps you manage stress and turn it into success.

- Sport Psychology helps you handle the paradox of success: An issue that every athlete faces at some time is the paradox of success. As you become more successful, there are more pressures and more distractions pulling at you. Sport psychology helps you address these, stay focused, and helps you continue to sustain your best performances.

Sports Hypnosis

Sports hypnosis refers to the use of hypnotherapy with athletes in order to enhance sporting performance. Hypnosis in sports has therapeutic and performance-enhancing functions. The mental state of athletes during training and competition is said to impact performance. Hypnosis is a form of mental training and can therefore contribute to enhancing athletic execution. Sports hypnosis is used by athletes, coaches and psychologists.

Hypnosis has been used in various professions including dentistry, medicine, psychotherapy and sports, as a performance enhancement tool. Sports hypnosis incorporates cognitive and sports science methodologies. Hypnosis in sports therefore overlaps with areas such as biomechanics, nutrition, physiology and sports psychology. Generally sports hypnosis is studied within the field of sports psychology, which examines the impact of psychological variables on athletes' performance. While sports psychology began to be studied around the 1920s, the study and use of hypnosis was not documented until the 1950s. Members of the Russian Olympic team are said to have made use of hypnosis as a performance-enhancing tool around this time.

Application

Although not referred to as hypnosis, professional athletes and teams have used an approach called guided imagery, which is much similar to techniques used in sports hypnosis.

Hypnosis is one of several techniques that athletes may employ to accomplish their sporting goals and it is equally beneficial to coaches as well as athletes. Hypnosis may do for the mind what physical activity does for the body of an athlete. The theory behind sports hypnosis is that relaxation is key to improved sporting performance and athletes may perform better if they are able to relax mentally and focus on the task at hand. Hypnosis may help athletes attain relaxation during practise and competition. Hypnosis may also help to control anxiety and manage stress in athletes. Athletes may develop auto-response to preestablished stimuli which is geared towards achieving optimal performance levels. Sports Hypnosis can also eliminate phobic responses, such as 'Trigger Freeze' in the Clay Pigeon Shooter, 'Target Panic' in the Archer and Fears of further injury in sports people following injury.

The impact of hypnosis on various aspects of sporting performance has been studied. Research has studied the role of hypnosis in enhancing basketball skills, on flow-state and golf-putting performance, its impact on long-distance runners, on archery performance and on flow states and short-serve in badminton.

The use of hypnosis in sports offers the following potential benefits that may help athletes handle personal challenges that would otherwise negatively affect sporting performance. Hypnosis:

- Helps to reinforce established sporting goals.
- Aids athletes to better handle nervousness.
- Contributes to relaxation.
- Facilitates stress management.
- Increases concentration.
- Eliminates sports phobia responses.
- Provides the ability to eliminate distractions.
- Assists in controlling pain.
- Increases performance motivation.
- Improves bodily awareness.

CONCONI TEST

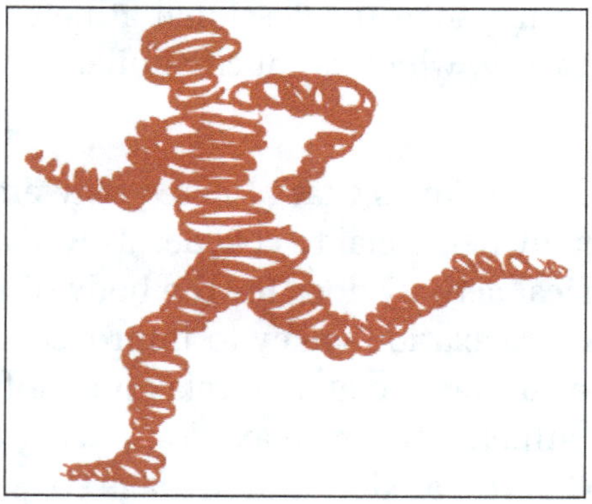

The Conconi Test was first described by Italian Sport Scientist Francesco Conconi in 1982 (Conconi et al. 1982). It is a relatively simple field test which measures the heart rate at different predefined intensity levels, which can be used to estimate Anaerobic Threshold, a point at which the body predominately uses the anaerobic energy system. It is also known as the ramp test.

- Purpose: To determine the heart rate at the anaerobic threshold for setting training zones.

- Equipment required: Stopwatch, heart rate monitor (with recording and recall function), running track or exercise equipment.
- Pre-test: Explain the test procedures to the subject. Perform screening of health risks and obtain informed consent. Prepare forms and record basic information such as age, height, body weight, gender, test conditions.
- Procedure: This test can be conducted on any equipment or during any exercise mode. Start at an easy pace, then at pre-determined intervals increase the workload. Record your heart rate at the end of each speed/workload level. Continue exercising until exhaustion.
- Scoring: Plot the heart rate over speed/workload as a graph. Connect the points with a line. Initially the heart rate and workload graph should be linear. At a high intensity, the point where the line bends corresponds to your anaerobic threshold. Record your heart rate and workload at this point on the graph.
- Accuracy: This test assumes that the anaerobic threshold is related to a deflection point on the heart rate/intensity graph. Subsequent studies have found that the deflection point in heart rate only occurs in a certain individuals and that when it does, it significantly overestimates directly measured lactate threshold.
- Target population: Endurance athletes (middle/long distance runners, cyclists, triathletes, rowers)
- Comments: Even if the anaerobic threshold level is not an accurate measure, you can use this test to look at improvements in fitness as your heart rate at each workload should decrease as you get fitter. You can also get a measure of your maximum heart rate from this test.

DIVING MEDICINE

Diving medicine, also called undersea and hyperbaric medicine (UHB), is the diagnosis, treatment and prevention of conditions caused by humans entering the undersea environment. It includes the effects on the body of pressure on gases, the diagnosis and treatment of conditions caused by marine hazards and how relationships of a diver's fitness to dive affect a diver's safety.

Hyperbaric medicine is a corollary field associated with diving, since recompression in a hyperbaric chamber is used as a treatment for two of the most significant diving-related illnesses, decompression sickness and arterial gas embolism.

Diving medicine deals with medical research on issues of diving, the prevention of diving disorders, treatment of diving accidents and diving fitness. The field includes the effect of breathing gases and their contaminants under high pressure on the human body and the relationship between the state of physical and psychological health of the diver and safety.

In diving accidents it is common for multiple disorders to occur together and interact with each other, both causatively and as complications.

Diving medicine is a branch of occupational medicine and sports medicine, and an important part of diver education.

Range and Scope of Diving Medicine

The scope of diving medicine must necessarily include conditions that are specifically connected with the activity of diving, and not found in other contexts, but this categorization excludes almost everything, leaving only deep water blackout, isobaric counterdiffusion and high pressure nervous syndrome. A more useful grouping is conditions that are associated with exposure to variations of ambient pressure. These conditions are largely shared by aviation and space medicine. Further conditions associated with diving and other aquatic and outdoor activities are commonly included in books which are aimed at the diver, rather than the specialist medical practitioner, as they are useful background to diver first aid training.

The scope of knowledge necessary for a practitioner of diving medicine includes the medical conditions associated with diving and their treatment, physics and physiology relating to the underwater and pressurised environment, the standard operating procedures and equipment used by divers which can influence the development and management of these conditions, and the specialised equipment used for treatment.

Scope of knowledge for Diving Medicine

The ECHM-EDTC Educational and Training Standards for Diving and Hyperbaric Medicine (2011) specify the following scope of knowledge for Diving Medicine:

<table>
<tr>
<td>

- Physiology and pathology of diving and hyperbaric exposure.
    - Hyperbaric physics
    - Diving related physiology
    - Hyperbaric pathophysiology of immersion
    - Pathophysiology of decompression
    - A brief introduction to acute dysbaric disorders
    - Chronic dysbaric disorders
    - Hyperbaric oxygen therapy basis - Physiology and pathology

</td>
<td>

- Fitness to dive
    - Fitness to dive criteria and contraindications for divers, compressed air workers and HBOT chamber personnel
    - Fitness to dive assessment
    - Fitness to dive standards (professional and recreational)
- Diving accidents
    - Diving incidents and accidents
    - Emergency medical support with no chamber on site

</td>
</tr>
</table>

- Oxygen toxicity
- Pressure and inert gas effects
  - Nitrogen narcosis
  - High pressure neurological syndrome
- Medication under pressure
- Non-dysbaric diving pathologies

- Diving technology and safety
  - Basic safety planning
  - Compressed air work
  - Diving procedures
    - Wet bells and stages
    - Scuba diving on air and mixed gas
    - Surface supplied diving
    - Standard diving (copper helmet)
    - Rebreather diving (semi-closed and closed circuit)
    - Other diving procedures
  - Characteristics of various divers
  - Diving equipment as used to c.50m and Chambers
  - Diving tables and computers
  - Regulations and standards for diving
  - Saturation diving
    - Saturation mode
    - Physiology of deep exposure
    - Compression
    - At depth in a living chamber
    - Bell excursions
    - Barotrauma: ENT; dental; cutaneous, conjunctival, etc.
    - Physical injuries
  - Decompression illness
    - Pathophysiological basis and mechanisms of DCI
    - Differential diagnosis of decompression illness
    - Management of decompression incidents at the surface
    - Immediate management, recompression tables and strategies
  - Rehabilitation of disabled divers
  - Diving accident investigation
- Clinical HBO
  - Recompression chamber

Scope of Knowledge for Hyperbaric Medicine

The ECHM-EDTC Educational and Training Standards for Diving and Hyperbaric Medicine (2011) specify the following scope of knowledge for Hyperbaric Medicine additional to that for Diving medicine:

- Physiology and pathology of diving and hyperbaric exposure.
  - HBO-Basics - effects of hyperbaric oxygen - physiology and pathology.

- Clinical HBO.
  - Chamber technique (multiplace, monoplace, transport chambers, wet recompression).
  - Mandatory indications.
  - HBO Recommended indications.
  - HBO Experimental and anecdotal indications.
  - HBO Data collection / statistics / evaluation.
  - HBO General basic treatment (nursing).
  - HBO Diagnostic, monitoring and therapeutic devices in chambers.
  - Risk assessment, incidents monitoring and safety plan in HBO chambers.
  - HBO Safety regulations.

Diagnostics

The signs and symptoms of diving disorders may present during a dive, on surfacing, or up to several hours after a dive. Divers have to breathe a gas which is at the same pressure as their surroundings, which can be much greater than on the surface. The ambient pressure underwater increases by 1 standard atmosphere (100 kPa) for every 10 metres (33 ft) of depth.

The principal conditions are: decompression illness (which covers decompression sickness and arterial gas embolism); nitrogen narcosis; high pressure nervous syndrome; oxygen toxicity; and pulmonary barotrauma (burst lung). Although some of these may occur in other settings, they are of particular concern during diving activities.

The disorders are caused by breathing gas at the high pressures encountered at depth, and divers will often breathe a gas mixture different from air to mitigate these effects. Nitrox, which contains more oxygen and less nitrogen is commonly used as a breathing gas to reduce the risk of decompression sickness at recreational depths (up to about 40 metres (130 ft)). Helium may be added to reduce the amount of nitrogen and oxygen in the gas mixture when diving deeper, to reduce the effects of narcosis and to avoid the risk of oxygen toxicity. This is complicated at depths beyond about 150 metres (500 ft), because a helium–oxygen mixture (heliox) then causes high pressure nervous syndrome. More exotic mixtures such as hydreliox, a hydrogen–helium–oxygen mixture, are used at extreme depths to counteract this.

Decompression Sickness

Decompression sickness (DCS) occurs when gas, which has been breathed under high pressure and dissolved into the body tissues, forms bubbles as the pressure is reduced on ascent from a dive. The results may range from pain in the joints where the bubbles form to blockage of an artery leading to damage to the nervous system, paralysis or death. While bubbles can form anywhere in the body, DCS is most frequently observed in the shoulders, elbows, knees, and ankles. Joint pain occurs in about 90% of DCS cases reported to the U.S. Navy, with neurological symptoms and skin manifestations each present in 10% to 15% of cases. Pulmonary DCS is very rare in divers.

Pulmonary Barotrauma and Arterial Gas Embolism

If the breathing gas in a diver's lungs cannot freely escape during an ascent, the lungs may be expanded beyond their compliance, and the lung tissues may rupture, causing pulmonary barotrauma (PBT). The gas may then enter the arterial circulation producing arterial gas embolism (AGE), with effects similar to severe decompression sickness. Gas bubbles within the arterial circulation can block the supply of blood to any part of the body, including the brain, and can therefore manifest a vast variety of symptoms.

Nitrogen Narcosis

Nitrogen narcosis is caused by the pressure of dissolved gas in the body and produces impairment to the nervous system. This results in alteration to thought processes and a decrease in the diver's ability to make judgements or calculations. It can also decrease motor skills, and worsen performance in tasks requiring manual dexterity. As depth increases, so does the pressure and hence the severity of the narcosis. The effects may vary widely from individual to individual, and from day to day for the same diver. Because of the perception-altering effects of narcosis, a diver may not be aware of the symptoms, but studies have shown that impairment occurs nevertheless.

High Pressure Nervous Syndrome

Helium is the least narcotic of all gases, and divers may use breathing mixtures containing a proportion of helium for dives exceeding about 40 metres (130 ft) deep. In the 1960s it was expected that helium narcosis would begin to become apparent at depths of 300 metres (1,000 ft). However, it was found that different symptoms, such as tremors, occurred at shallower depths around 150 metres (500 ft). This became known as high pressure nervous syndrome, and its effects are found to result from both the absolute depth and the speed of descent. Although the effects vary from person to person, they are stable and reproducible for the individual.

Oxygen Toxicity

Although oxygen is essential to life, in concentrations significantly greater than normal it becomes toxic, overcoming the body's natural defences (antioxidants), and causing cell death in any part of the body. The lungs and brain are particularly affected by high partial pressures of oxygen, such as are encountered in diving. The body can tolerate partial pressures of oxygen around 0.5 bars (50 kPa; 7.3 psi) indefinitely, and up to 1.4 bars (140 kPa; 20 psi) for many hours, but higher partial pressures rapidly increase the chance of the most dangerous effect of oxygen toxicity, a convulsion resembling an epileptic seizure. Susceptibility to oxygen toxicity varies dramatically from person to person, and to a smaller extent from day to day for the same diver. Prior to convulsion, several symptoms may be present – most distinctly that of an aura.

Treatments

Treatment of diving disorders depends on the specific disorder or combination of disorders, but two treatments are commonly associated with first aid and definitive treatment where diving is involved. These are first aid oxygen administration at high concentration, which is seldom contraindicated, and generally recommended as a default option in diving accidents where there is any significant probability of hypoxia, and hyperbaric oxygen therapy, which is the definitive treatment for most incidences of decompression illness. Hyperbaric treatment using other breathing gases is also used for treatment of decompression sickness if HBO is inadequate.

Oxygen Therapy

The administration of oxygen as a medical intervention is common in diving medicine, both for first aid and for longer term treatment. Normobaric oxygen administration at the highest available concentration is frequently used as first aid for any diving injury that may involve inert gas bubble formation in the tissues. There is epidemiological support for its use from a statistical study of cases recorded in a long term database.

Recompression and Hyperbaric Oxygen Therapy

Recompression treatment in a hyperbaric chamber was initially used as a life-saving tool to treat decompression sickness in caisson workers and divers who stayed too long at depth and developed decompression sickness. Now, it is a highly specialized treatment modality that has been found to be effective in the treatment of many conditions where the administration of oxygen under pressure has been found to be beneficial. Studies have shown it to be quite effective in some 13 indications approved by the Undersea and Hyperbaric Medical Society.

Hyperbaric oxygen treatment is generally preferred when effective, as it is usually a more efficient and lower risk method of reducing symptoms of decompression illness, but in some cases recompression to pressures where oxygen toxicity is unacceptable may be required to eliminate the bubbles in the tissues in severe cases of decompression illness.

Education and Registration of Practitioners

Specialist training in underwater and hyperbaric medicine is available from several institutions, and registration is possible both with professional associations and governmental registries.

Education

NOAA/UHMS Physicians Training Course in Diving Medicine

This course has been presented since 1977, and has been influenced by internationally accepted training objectives recommended by the Diving Medical Advisory Committee, the European Diving Technology Committee, and the European Committee for Hyperbaric Medicine. The course is designed for qualified medical practitioners, but may be useful to others who work in the field of diving safety and operations. The course is to train physicians to recognize and treat diving medical emergencies. Subject matter includes:

- Basic physics and physiology of the hyperbaric environment:
  - The laws and principles;
  - The differences between hyperbaric and hypobaric pressure;
  - Hyperbaric gases and their effects under pressure;
  - Links between the physiological effects of the hyperbaric environment and the pathology of the disease.
- Basic decompression theory:
  - Historical development to current concepts;
  - Factors affecting decompression safety including acceptable risks and thermal issues;
  - Distinguish decompression sickness from barotrauma and arterial gas embolism.
- Dive computer theories and types, and comparison to dive tables;
- Introduction to commercial diving and comparison to recreational and technical diving, including differences in procedures, equipment, and diver categories;
- The clinical application of hyperbaric oxygen therapy and the treatment tables used;
- Participation in surface-supplied diving operation and hyperbaric chamber operations;
- Components, types, operational and safety hazards associated with hyperbaric chambers;

- Diving-related conditions resulting from the effects of long-term effects of diving, flying after diving, altitude, thermal conditions, age and gender;
- Neurologic assessment on a diver with signs and/or symptoms of DCI.
- Medical and fitness standards for diving, including:
    - Contraindications for both commercial and recreational divers;
    - Differences in medical standards for recreational versus occupational diving communities;
    - Legal implications for approving and denying fitness to dive in an occupational setting;
    - Approaches for determining the safety of prescription and OTC medications used by divers.

Fellowship in Undersea and Hyperbaric Medicine

The Accreditation Council for Graduate Medical Education (ACGME) and the American Osteopathic Association (AOA) offer 12 month programs in undersea and hyperbaric medicine associated with ACGME or AOA accredited programs in emergency medicine, family medicine, internal medicine, occupational medicine, preventive medicine, or anesthesiology.

ECHM-EDTC Educational and Training Standards for Physicians in Diving and Hyperbaric Medicine

The standard drawn up jointly by the European Committee for Hyperbaric Medicine and the European Diving Technical Committee defines job descriptions for several levels of diving and hyperbaric physician: Education and assessment to these standards may be provided by institutions of higher education under the leadership of a Level 3 Hyperbaric Medicine Expert as defined below. Certificates of competence may be issued by a nationally accredited institution or an internationally acknowledged agency, and periodic recertification is required.

Level 1: Medical Examiner of Divers (MED) minimum 28 teaching hours-

- The MED must be competent to perform the assessments of medical fitness to dive of occupational and recreational divers and compressed air workers, except the assessment of medical fitness to resume diving after major decompression incidents.

Level 2D: *Diving Medicine Physician* (DMP) minimum 80 teaching hours-

- A DMP must be competent to perform the initial and all other assessments of medical fitness to dive of working and recreational divers or compressed air workers, and manage diving accidents and advise diving contractors and others on diving medicine and physiology (with the backup of a diving medical expert or consultant).

- A DMP should have knowledge in relevant aspects of occupational health, but is not required to be a certified specialist in occupational medicine.
- A DMP should have certified skills and basic practical experience in assessment of medical fitness to dive, management of diving accidents, safety planning for professional diving operations, advanced life support, acute trauma care and general wound care.

Level 2H: Hyperbaric Medicine Physician (HMP) minimum 120 teaching hours-

- An HMP will be responsible for hyperbaric treatment sessions (with the backup of a hyperbaric medicine expert or consultant).
- An HMP should have appropriate experience in anaesthesia and intensive care in order to manage the HBO patients, but is not required to be a certified specialist in anaesthesia and intensive care.
- An HMP must be competent to assess and manage clinical patients for hyperbaric oxygen therapy treatment.

Level 3: Hyperbaric medicine expert or consultant (hyperbaric and diving medicine) is a physician who has been assessed as competent to-

- Manage a hyperbaric facility (HBO centre) or the medical and physiological aspects of complex diving activities.
- Manage research programs on diving medicine.
- Supervise a team of HBO doctors and personnel, health professionals and others.
- Teach relevant aspects of hyperbaric medicine and physiology to all members of staff.

Gesellschaft für Tauch- und Überdruckmedizin e. V.

Society for Diving and Hyperbaric medicine: German standards for education and assessment of diving medical practitioners are similar to the ECHM-EDTC Standards and are controlled by the Gesellschaft für Tauch- und Überdruckmedizin e. V. They include Medical Examiner of Divers, Diving Medicine Physician, Hyperbaric Medicine Physician, Chief Hyperbaric Medicine Physician and Hyperbaric Medicine Consultant.

Schweizerische Gesellschaft für Unterwasser- und Hyperbarmedizin

Swiss Society for underwater and hyperbaric medicine: Swiss standards for education and assessment of diving medical practitioners are controlled by the Schweizerische

Gesellschaft für Unterwasser- und Hyperbarmedizin. They include Medical Examiner of Divers, Diving Medicine Physician and Hyperbaric Medicine Physician.

Österreichische Gesellschaft für Tauch- und Hyperbarmedizin

Austrian Society for Diving and Hyperbaric medicine: Austrian standards for education and assessment of diving medical practitioners are controlled by the Österreichische Gesellschaft für Tauch- und Hyperbarmedizin They include Medical Examiner of Divers, Diving Medicine Physician, Hyperbaric Medicine Physician, Chief Hyperbaric Medicine Physician and Hyperbaric Medicine Consultant.

Registration

The American Medical Association recognises the sub-speciality Undersea and Hyperbaric Medicine held by someone who is already Board Certified in some other speciality.

The South African Department of Labour registers two levels of *Diving Medical Practitioner*. Level 1 is qualified to conduct annual examinations and certification of medical fitness to dive, on commercial divers (equivalent to ECHM-EDTC Level 1. Medical Examiner of Divers), and Level 2 is qualified to provide medical advice to a diving contractor and hyperbaric treatment for diving injuries.

Australia has a four tier system: In 2007 there was no recognised equivalence with the European standard.

- GPs completing the first tier four- to five-day course on how to examine divers for 'fitness to dive' can then add their names to the SPUMS Diving Doctors List
- GPs completing the second tier two-week diving medicine courses provided by the Royal Australian Navy and the Royal Adelaide Hospital, or the two-week course in Diving and Hyperbaric Medicine provided by the ANZ Hyperbaric Medicine Group, qualify to do commercial-diving medicals.
- The third tier is the SPUMS Diploma in Diving and Hyperbaric Medicine. The candidate must attend a two-week course, write a dissertation related to DHM and have the equivalent of six months' full-time experience working in a hyperbaric medicine unit.
- The fourth tier is the Certificate in Diving and Hyperbaric Medicine from the ANZ College of Anaesthetists.

Training of Divers and Support Staff in Relevant First Aid

Divers

A basic knowledge understanding of the causes, symptoms and first aid treatment of diving related disorders is part of the basic training for most recreational and professional divers, both to help the diver avoid the disorders, and to allow appropriate action in case of an incident resulting in injury.

Recreational Divers

A recreational diver has the same duty of care to other divers as any ordinary member of the public, and therefore there is no obligation to train recreational divers in first aid or other medical skills. Nevertheless, first aid is training is recommended by most, if not all, recreational diver training agencies.

Recreational diving instructors and divemasters, on the other hand, are to a greater or lesser extent responsible for the safety of divers under their guidance, and therefore are generally required to be trained and certified to some level of rescue and first aid competence, as defined in the relevant training standards of the certifying body. In many cases this includes certification in Cardiopulmonary resuscitation and Oxygen administration for diving accidents.

Professional Divers

Professional divers usually operate as members of a team with a duty of care for other members of the team. Divers are expected to act as standby divers for other members of the team and the duties of a standby diver include rescue attempts if the working diver gets into difficulties. Consequently, professional divers are generally required to be trained in rescue procedures appropriate to the modes of diving they are certified in, and to administer first aid in emergencies. The specific training, competence and registration for these skills varies, and may be specified by state or national legislation or by industry codes of practice.

Diving supervisors have a similar duty of care, and as they are responsible for operational planning and safety, generally are also expected to manage emergency procedures, including the first aid that may be required. The level of first aid training, competence and certification will generally take this into account.

- In South Africa, registered commercial and scientific divers must hold current certification in first aid at the national Level 1, with additional training in oxygen administration for diving accidents, and registered diving supervisors must hold Level 2 first aid certification.
- Offshore diving contractors frequently follow the IMCA recommendations.

Diver Medic

A diver medic or diving medical technician (DMT) is a member of a dive team who is trained in advanced first aid. A Diver Medic recognised by IMCA must be capable of administering First Aid and emergency treatment, and carrying out the directions of a doctor pending the arrival of more skilled medical aid, and therefore must be able to effectively communicate with a doctor who is not on site, and be familiar with diving procedures and compression chamber operation. The Diver Medic must also be able to assist the diving supervisor with decompression procedures provide advice as to when more specialised medical help should be requested, and must be fit to provide treatment in a hyperbaric chamber in an emergency, and must therefore hold a valid certificate of medical fitness to dive.

Training standards for Diver Medic are described in the IMCA Scheme for Recognition of Diver Medic Training.

ORTHOPEDIC SPORTS MEDICINE

Orthopedic sports medicine is a subspecialty of Orthopedics that focuses on managing pathological conditions of the musculoskeletal system arising from sports practice. When dealing with athletes, timing is the most difficult issue to face. Typically, athletes aim to return to play as soon as possible and at the pre-injury level. This means that management should be optimized to combine the need for prompt return to sport and to the biologic healing time of the musculo-skeletal. This poses a great challenge to sport medicine surgeons, who need to follow with attention to the latest scientific evidence to offer their patients the best available treatment options. We briefly review the most commonly performed orthopedic sports medicine procedures, outlining the presently available scientific evidence on their indications and outcomes.

About 11 athletes out of 100 participating in the Olympic Games will face an injury, based on the data from the last three editions. Although the highest incidence occurs in contact sports, such as football, American football, hockey, and martial arts, some of the non-contact sports as athletics are equally affected by high rates of injuries. Looking again at the Olympic Games data, about half of the injuries involves the lower limb, 20% the upper limb, while head, neck, and trunk account all together for 25%. About a quarter of all the injuries are overuse injuries, which are more likely to occur in non-contact sports. Regardless of whether an injury is acute or overuse, the main issue in dealing with athletes is timing. The deeply engrained strong desire to return to play, within the shortest time, is the main challenge for sport medicine surgeons and drives treatment choices.

Lower Limb

Knee

Meniscal injuries: Although meniscal injuries are mainly encountered in athletes involved in pivoting maneuvers, even low-impact sports such as swimming have been plagued by meniscal lesions. Meniscal injuries are one of the most common musculo-skeletal issues and one of the most common orthopedic surgery performed worldwide. Vertical peripheral longitudinal tears as well as root tears should be repaired, leading to superior outcomes in terms of symptoms, function, return to play, and cartilage preservation compared to meniscectomy. In more recent years, there is an increasing body of evidence in favor of repairing horizontal tears, especially in the young patient. Return to sports after meniscus repair for high-level athletes (basketball, American football, baseball) varies between 80 and 90%. However, studies on meniscal repair in athletes have found that up to one third of the patients underwent reoperation for pain. Concerning the surgical technique of a meniscal repair, there is general agreement to start the procedure performing a debridement and abrasion of the meniscal lesion walls to favor local bleeding, and with regard to the suture technique, vertical or horizontal sutures are recommended, performed either with all-inside, inside-out or outside-in techniques, since no superiority have been demonstrated of one technique over the others. However, it has been demonstrated that vertical suturing configuration has superior load to failure values compared to a horizontal configuration. Usually, all-inside sutures are used on the far posterior segments, and inside-out for the middle and anterior meniscal segments. Alvarez-Diaz et al., in a case-series on 29 competitive football players, reported that 26 (89.6%) were able to return to play at the same level of competition at a mean of 4.3 months after surgery.

Anterior Cruciate Ligament Injury

Anterior cruciate ligament (ACL) tears, accounting for about 200,000 injuries per year in the USA, may compromise knee stability and affect negatively sports activity. Although most of the ACL tears result from a non-contact injury, lesions during contrasts in sports such as American football, rugby, or hockey are frequent as well.

Many risk factors have been identified for ACL tear. Some depend on bone morphology (narrower intercondylar notch widths, smaller notch width index, and increased tibial slopes), some others on hormones and gender. Recently, biomechanical factors such as limited hip internal rotation have been associated to ACL tear injury. Conservative management of ACL tears can produce acceptable results, but in athletes, surgical reconstruction is usually preferred. The main advantage of ACL reconstruction (ACLR) is to restore knee stability what will eventually help to prevent secondary injury to menisci and articular cartilage. Different techniques are used to perform ACLR. Transtibial independent drilling (through the antero-medial portal) and the outside-in techniques are the most commonly used ones. A systematic review showed that independent drilling is more likely to lead to better biomechanical and functional outcomes compared to transtibial technique, although no clear clinical evidences support its superiority. Outside-in drilling has the advantages of unconstrained tunnels placement, but it needs two incisions. Single- or double-bundle graft reconstructions have been proposed. Biomechanical studies favored double-bundle graft in terms of rotational stability; however, no clinical superiority has been shown.

Concerning the graft, it is possible to identify three main categories: autograft, allograft, and synthetic graft. Synthetic graft showed high failure rate, although newer synthetic grafts seem, in the short term, more promising than the older ones.

Allografts are expensive; there is a risk for infections transmission, delayed incorporation, and late failure. Therefore, especially for young athletic individuals, the choice falls on autografts: Bone patellar tendon bone (BPTB), hamstrings, and less commonly quadriceps tendon. There is a huge debate on what is better between patellar tendon and hamstring, and no definitive superiority has been shown. BPTB grafts ensure greater post-operative knee stability but exhibit a higher complication rate. On the contrary, hamstring autograft, for which revision surgery is most frequently required, is often associated with post-operative antero-posterior knee laxity, particularly in females. However, despite all the great efforts trying to improve ACL reconstruction, the rate of patients who return to sports ranges between 63 and 92%. This trend confirms the importance of psychological factor and neuromuscular focused rehabilitation as essential elements in determining the return to play rat.

Posterior Cruciate Ligament Injury

Isolate posterior cruciate ligament (PCL) injury has an incidence that ranges between 3 and 44% after acute trauma to the knee. A PCL injury is often part of complex knee injuries, associated respectively in 46, 31, and 62% of cases, to ACL tears, medial collateral ligament (MCL) injury, and posterolateral corner injuries. Isolated PCL injuries in the knees with reduced joint laxity and absence of other peripheral lesion are generally managed conservatively even in athletes, with satisfactory subjective results, and return to sport at the same level in about 50% of cases. In patients with PCL injuries managed conservatively, 41% of the subjects at 14-year follow-up develop early osteoarthritis, with progressive reduction of joint function. Surgical treatment can be performed to optimize joint function. After surgery, competitive sports are practiced again by 67% of the subjects and high functional demand sports by 26%. Clinical outcomes show no differences between single- and double-bundle reconstruction techniques at approximately 30 months of follow-up. However, double-bundle PCL reconstruction mainly improves objective measurement of knee stability.

Hip

Femoroacetabular Impingement

Femoroacetabular impingement (FAI) is a common cause of hip and groin pain in young active people and athletes. FAI initially causes chondral lesions and labral tears and, subsequently, early arthritis. Arthroscopic surgery is undertaken in subjects refractory to conservative management, involving targeted physiotherapy and oral anti-inflammatory drugs. Few studies reported data about surgical procedures, such as femoroplasty, acetabuloplasty, and labral reconstruction, in athletes, and they showed that arthroscopic surgery is effective in terms of both clinical and functional improvement and return to sport (87% of patients). Moreover, timing for arthroscopic treatment is essential; the length of athletic career was significantly affected by symptom duration before arthroscopic treatment in professional hockey players.

Achilles Tendon

Achilles tendinopathy is common in athletes, accounting for 6–17% of all injuries in running athletes. The etiology of tendinopaty is still not well understood, but multiple factors play a role in its pathophysiology. Pharmacological interventions currently lack for scientific evidences supporting their use, while conservative management of chronic midportion Achilles tendinopathy by eccentric exercises and extracorporeal shock waves therapy (ESWT) is strongly supported by several level I studies. Patients resistant to those conservative measures can undergo to high-volume image-guided injection, effective in relieving patients' symptoms and restore tendon function both in the short and long term. In non-insertional Achilles tendinopathy, minimally invasive multiple percutaneous longitudinal tenotomies are valid alternatives to more invasive procedures, at least in patients without evidence of paratendinopathy, unresponsive to 6 months of conservative management. This method leads to satisfactory outcomes in the long term and restores ankle function. Given the renowned complications in terms of infections and difficult wound healing, in most recent years, tendoscopy has been proposed, with satisfactory outcomes, as an alternative method to open surgery, including debridement alone or debridement associated to flexor halluces longus tendon transfer.

Eccentric exercises for insertional Achilles tendinopaty did not show excellent outcomes, while ESWT did better according to a quite recent systematic review. For those patients not responding to conservative measures, surgery is indicated in order to debride the tendinopathic tissue and/or to excise the calcaneal bony prominence, with or without tendon detachment and subsequent fixation to calcaneus tuberosity. Surgical management of insertional Achilles tendinopathy is indicated after failure of 3- to 6-month period of nonsurgical management. Thorough debridement is necessary, and this leads often to a near to complete detachment of the tendon's insertion. Therefore, repair with two anchors is recommended; indeed, it is associated with good to excellent results. Outcomes from surgery can be satisfactory, but prolonged rehabilitation is necessary.

Ankle

Lateral Ankle Ligaments

Ankle sprains are common, especially in team sports. They account for up to 40% of all athletic injuries, and 29% of American football injuries can be attributed to ankle injuries. The most common pattern of injury is forefoot adduction, hindfoot inversion, with the tibia externally rotated and the ankle in plantar flexion. This mechanism leads to tears to one or more of the lateral ligaments of the ankle. Up to 70% of the sprains involve the anterior talo-fibular ligament (ATFL) alone. More than 50% of the ankle sprains do not come to medical attention. Patients with ankle sprain grade I and II, accounting for greatest part, will benefit from the use of RICE (rest, ice [cryotherapy], compression, and elevation). Grade III has a less standardized management. Some authors have proposed surgical repair for the acute grade III lesion, but many others have reported discouraging outcomes following acute repair in favor of functional treatment.

Chronic ankle instability is defined as the condition of symptomatic ankle instability following an acute ankle sprain managed with conservative measure.

Surgical management of the lateral ligaments of the ankle can be performed with an anatomic reconstruction (the Brostrom-Gould technique) or by several techniques in which a tendon graft, either autograft or allograft, reinforces the local tissue. A recent comparison of lateral anatomic ankle repair (Brostrom-Gould) to allograft reconstruction showed that no revision was needed in patients from both groups, and no significant differences between groups in terms of function and patients' satisfaction were found.

Allografts showed good to excellent results in up to 85% of cases, and they should be considered when multiple ligaments are involved, such as calcaneofibular ligament (CFL) other than ATFL.

At the time of surgical repair of ankle lateral ligaments, it is highly recommended to perform an ankle arthroscopy, since this will allow looking for intrarticular lesions.

Recently, different minimally invasive techniques have been proposed for chronic ankle instability (arthroscopic repair, non-arthroscopic minimally invasive repair, arthroscopic reconstruction, and non-arthroscopic minimally invasive reconstruction). However, there is still a lack for high-level evidences to support their use in daily clinical practice.

Ankle Osteochondral Lesions

About 50% of acute ankle sprain leads to chondral lesions of the talus (OCL), causing persisting pain despite conservative or surgical treatment. Most of the OCL are central-lateral (49%) and follow an inversion ankle sprain. Those kinds of lesions respond poorly to conservative measures. In the acute setting, arthroscopic debridement with excision of the loose OCL is usually indicated for lesions smaller than 1 cm^2. Fragment fixation using bioabsorbable screws is advised for wider lesion.

Chronic OCLs are classified in five types according to Loomer et al. Type I and II lesions can be addressed by retrograde drilling, a technique that aims to bone marrow stimulation.Type III and IV lesions can be addressed with satisfactory outcomes either by excision or curettage. Finally, type V, a cystic lesion, is usually bone grafted or filled using osteochondral plugs (mosaicplasty).

Spine

Disc Herniation and Disc Degeneration Disease

Injuries of the cervical spine frequently affect athletes who practice contact sports and represent 44.7% of all American football-related spinal injuries. In patients with diagnosis of cervical disc herniations, surgical indications are persistent symptoms, evidence of spinal cord compression on MRI and cervical myelopathy. However, drug (such as anti-inflammatory medications) and physical therapy (strengthening exercises) remains the first-line treatment and produces a higher rate of return to sport if compared with surgical treatment. Furthermore, contact sports are contraindicated in patients who underwent multilevel anterior cervical discectomy and fusion (ACDF) or with cervical myelopathy, residual pain, or muscle weakness.

Low back pain, reported by 75% of elite athletes, is frequent in athletes of all levels. In addition to genetic and anatomic factors, the incidence of lumbar disc degeneration is justified by an abnormal and increased load on the lumbar spine arising from sports activity practiced over the years, which, in the long term, leads to early disc degeneration. Similar to the upper spine levels, in lumbar pathology, the first approach is rehabilitation focused on restoring range of motion and muscular strengthening. Surgery is reserved to symptomatic patients non-responsive to non-operative treatment with imaging evidence of spinal cord compression. Lumbar disc herniation successfully receives non-operative treatment in 90% of patients. Professional athletes who underwent surgery, both total disc replacement or discectomy and fusion, experience significant improvement of symptoms in a high percentage of cases and about 95% of patients return to sport without significant differences with previous sports performances. Lumbar discectomy offers variable results according to the type of sport practiced by professional athletes. Satisfactory outcomes and high rates of return to sport can be found in American football players. On the contrary, baseball players who underwent surgery had a shorter career compared to colleagues with the same diagnosis but treated conservatively. This heterogeneity highlights the importance of load forces as causes of lumbar hernia and possible post-surgical recurrence. Treatment should be guided by surgeon experience and set on athlete's functional requirements.

Upper Limb

Shoulder

In athletes, shoulder injuries commonly involve rotator cuff tendons and the labrum.

- Superior labrum anterior to posterior (SLAP) lesions.

Snyder reported an incidence of SLAP lesions ranging from 4.8 to 6.9%. The injury mechanism is usually overhead activity that determines a contact between the articular side of the supraspinatus tendon and the postero-superior glenoid labrum.

The first line of treatment can be conservative, mainly aiming to scapula stabilization, rotator cuff strengthening, and stretching of the postero-inferior capsule. Indeed, an excessive loss of glenohumeral internal rotation (GIRD) is common in overhead athletes.

Surgical indication depends on several factors, such as the kind of lesion, the patient's age, level of activity, and the previous non-operative management. Type II SLAPs are the most common. They present complete detachment of the superior labrum and the biceps anchor from the superior glenoid tubercle. Repairing the lesion in older patients (>40 years old) showed higher rate of unsatisfactory outcomes and surgical revision. In this instance, the tendon of the long head of the biceps can undergo either a tenodesis or a tenotomy. In young active athletes, the lesion should be repaired. However, this is the most challenging type of lesion: its repair can result in a stiff shoulder, and return to play at the pre-injury level cannot be guaranteed. When choosing the treatment method, in type II lesion, it is of paramount to take into account the patient's type and level of activity. Recent evidences showed that biceps suprapectoral or subpectoral tenodesis is preferable over SLAP repair in young patients practicing overhead activity. Type I lesions are characterized by frying of the labrum, and therefore, the proposed surgical treatment is arthroscopic debridement. Type III lesions show a bucket handle tear of the labrum, while the biceps tendon is normal. For these lesions, resection of the unstable bucket handle tear is indicated. Type IV is a type III lesion with a longitudinal lesion of the biceps tendon, which may dislocate into the joint. When less than 30% of the tendon is torn, the lesion can be abraded together with the degenerated area of the labrum. If the lesion involves more than 30% of the biceps tendon, it will be repaired in young patients or excised in older ones.

Bankart Lesion

Anterior shoulder dislocation is common especially in contact athletes such as American football, ice hockey, and rugby players. The most common injury mechanism in athletes is abduction and external rotation of the arm by an externally rotating force. This injury mechanism generates a Bankart lesion where the antero-inferior capsule-labral complex is detached from the glenoid rim either alone or with a bony fragment (bony Bankart). In athletes, even after the first dislocation, non-operative treatment leads to a high recurrence rate.

Arthroscopic repair of the Bankart lesion has become more popular than open surgery, with similar reoperation and recurrence rate. Return to sport after arthroscopic Bankart repair is variable, going up to 95%. In bony Bankart lesions, following the new concept of glenoid track introduced by Itoi in 2007, there has been much debate on which is the best treatment to address both the humeral (Hill-Sachs) and the glenoid bony lesions. It is suggested to perform arthroscopic Bankart repair for patients with glenoid bone loss < 25% and on-track Hill-Sachs (HS). If the HS is off-track, a remplissage procedure is necessary to restore shoulder stability. When facing a glenoid bone loss > 25%, whether it is on-track or off-track HS, the Latarjet procedure is recommended.

Rotator Cuff Tears

Throwing athletes are at higher risk not only for labrum injuries but also for rotator cuff tears. In addition to the common cuff lesions, the throwing athletes show a higher incidence of partial-thickness articular-sided tears of the postero-superior portion of the cuff compared to the general population. This is secondary to the internal impingement syndrome, a phenomenon described by Jobe and Walch.

That syndrome is due to a conflict between the posterior glenoid rim and the postero-superior rotator cuff insertion on the greater tuberosity. Factors associated with this condition are recurring microtrauma, scapular diskynesis, and posterior capsule contracture with consequent loss of internal rotation.

Surgical options are taken into consideration when conservative measures have failed. In general, partial tears are repaired when the tear involves more than 50% of the tendon thickness; otherwise, the debridement alone is enough. However, it is controversial whether to repair partial lesions of the rotator cuff in a throwing athlete because of the difficulties of returning to play after a rotator cuff repair.

References

- Sports, graduate: apa.org, Retrieved 19 May, 2019
- Pates, John; Oliver, Rachael; Maynard, Ian (2001). "The effects of hypnosis on flow states and golf-putting performance". Journal of Applied Sport Psychology. 13 (4): 341–354. Citeseerx 10.1.1.523.3174. Doi:10.1080/104132001753226238
- Sports-medicine, science: britannica.com, Retrieved 15 January, 2019
- Hartman, Randy J. (2000-09-29). Shhh, Hypnotic Work in Progress: Twelve Case Histories in Clinical Hypnotherapy. ISBN 978-0595141883
- Sports-physiotherapy-and-rehabilitation, services: ssmc.sg, Retrieved 16 February, 2019
- Pates, John; Oliver, Rachael; Maynard, Ian (2001). "The effects of hypnosis on flow states and golf-putting performance". Journal of Applied Sport Psychology. 13 (4): 341–354. Citeseerx 10.1.1.523.3174. Doi:10.1080/104132001753226238
- Sport-physiotherapy, what-is-physiother: physiocanhelp.ca, Retrieved 17 March, 2019
- Staff (2005). "Swiss Underwater and Hyperbaric Medical Society" (in German). Lengnau: SUHMS Secretariat. Retrieved 12 March 2018
- Sports-chiropractic-the-athletes-secret-weapon, lake-forest-31004, lake-forest, California: the-joint.com, Retrieved 18 April, 2019

General Sports Injuries and their Treatment

CHAPTER 2

Injuries that occur during athletic activities, sports or exercise are called sports injuries. Ankle injury, knee injury, shin pain, patellar tendinitis, groin strain, Achilles tendon rupture, athletic heart syndrome, hamstring injuries and female athlete triad are some of the common sports injuries. This chapter has been carefully written to provide an easy understanding of these types of sports injuries and their treatment.

ANKLE INJURY

Sprains to the ankle are one of the most common sporting injuries. A sprain is defined as a tearing of the ligaments that connect bone to bone and help stabilise the joint.

Sports requiring jumping, turning and twisting movements such as basketball, volleyball, netball and football; and explosive changes of direction such as soccer, tennis and hockey are particularly vulnerable to ankle sprains.

Following an ankle sprain, the ankle joint may become unstable and take a long time to recover.

Anatomy

The ankle joint is a hinge joint formed between the tibia and fibula (bones of the lower leg) and the talus (a bone of the foot) and allows the foot to bend upwards (dorsiflexion) and downwards (plantarflexion). The joint also allows a small amount of rotation. Two bones of the foot, the talus and calcaneus (heel bone) connect to form the subtalar joint which allows the foot to rock side to side (inversion/eversion).

The joint's stability comes from the structural arrangement of the bones and the surrounding ligaments. Ligaments provide stability by preventing the amount of side to side movement. On the inside of the ankle (medial side), the joint is stabilised by a thick, strong fibrous ligament called the deltoid ligament. Sprains to the deltoid ligament (eversion sprains, foot twists outward) account for less than 20% of all ankle sprains.

On the outside of the ankle (lateral side), the joint is stabilised by three smaller ligaments; the anterior talofibular (at the front), the calcaneofibular (at the side) and the posterior talofibular (at the back). Sprains to any of these ligaments (inversion sprains, foot twists inward) account for more than 80% of all ankle sprains.

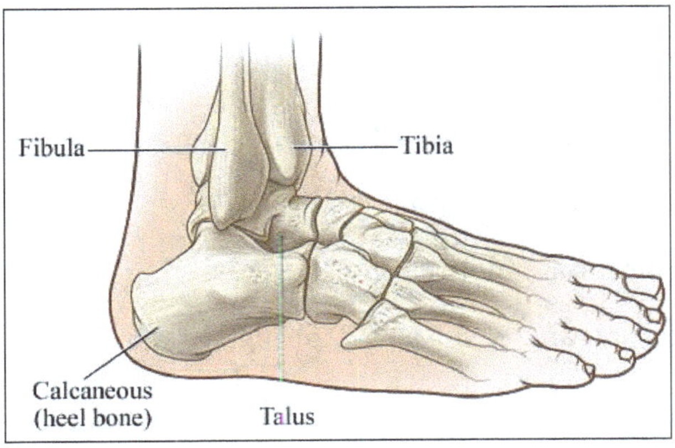

The most commonly injured ligament is the anterior talofibular. Injury to this ligament results in swelling and pain on the outside of the ankle. If the force is more severe, the calcaneofibular ligament is also damaged. The posterior talofibular ligament is less likely to be damaged. A complete tear of all ligaments may result in a dislocation of the ankle joint and an accompanying fracture.

Occasionally medial ligament injuries may be seen in conjunction with a lateral ligament injury.

The inferofebular ligament can also be injured. Injury to this ligament can be a cause of prolonged recovery from a sprain. Ligament sprains to the ankle joint may also involve the ligaments between the tibia and fibula bones. These injuries may involve a fracture, are often slower to recover, and may require surgery.

Risk

Acute ankle sprains result from a force being applied to the ankle joint which causes excessive range of movement at the joint. Players are immediately aware of the condition and may hear an audible 'snap' or 'pop', due to the tearing or stretching of the ligaments.

Proven Risk Factors

- Previous or existing ankle injury especially if poorly rehabilitated (biggest risk factor).
- Lack of strength and stability related to the ankle.
- Lack of, or extreme flexibility, in the ankle joint.
- Poor balance.

- Sudden change in direction (acceleration or deceleration).
- Increasing age of player.

Suspected Risk Factors

- Poor condition of the playing surface.
- Inappropriate, inadequate, or no warm-up.
- Wearing inappropriate footwear for the activity.
- Lack of external ankle support (taping, bracing) for previously injured ankles.

Prevention

- Undertaking training prior to competition to ensure readiness to play.
- Gradually increasing the intensity and duration of training.
- Undertaking flexibility, balance, stretching and strengthening exercises in weekly training programs.
- Including agility work in training programs so the ankle joint is capable of sustaining high acceleration forces and quick changes in direction.
- Allowing adequate recovery time between workouts or training sessions.
- Warming up to ensure surrounding muscles are ready to support the joint during activity.
- Wearing ankle taping or bracing especially for previously injured ankles.
- Wearing shoes appropriate to the sport that provide stability and support.
- Checking the training and playing area to ensure a flat and even surface.
- Drinking water before, during and after play.
- Avoiding activities that cause pain. If pain does occur, discontinuing the activity immediately and commencing RICER.

Signs and Symptoms

Sprains are graded on a scale of 1 to 3 (mild, moderate, and severe), depending on the degree of tearing to the ligaments. In most cases, x-rays are performed to rule out a fracture or dislocation.

Grade	Description
1 (mild)	• Minor tear • Minimal pain • Little of no joint instability • Mild pain with weight bearing activities • Slight loss of balance
2 (moderate)	• Some tearing of the ligament fibres • Moderate to severe pain • Moderate instability of the joint • Swelling and stiffness • Pain with weight bearing activities • Poor balance
3 (severe)	• Complete tear of the ligament • Severe pain followed by minimal pain • Gross instability of the joint • Severe swelling • Possible pain with weight bearing • Poor balance

Immediate Management

The immediate treatment of any soft tissue injury consists of the RICER protocol – rest, ice, compression, elevation and referral. RICE protocol should be followed for 48–72 hours. The aim is to reduce the bleeding and damage within the joint. The ankle should be rested in an elevated position with an ice pack applied for 20 minutes every two hours (never apply ice directly to the skin). A correctly sized compression bandage should be applied to limit bleeding and swelling in the joint.

The No HARM protocol should also be applied – no heat, no alcohol, no running or activity, and no massage. This will ensure decreased bleeding and swelling in the injured area.

A sports medicine professional should be seen as soon as possible after the injury to determine the extent of injury and to advise on treatment and rehabilitation. In evaluating the injury the sports medicine professional may order an x-ray or other testing to determine the extent of the injury.

Sprained Ankle Treatment

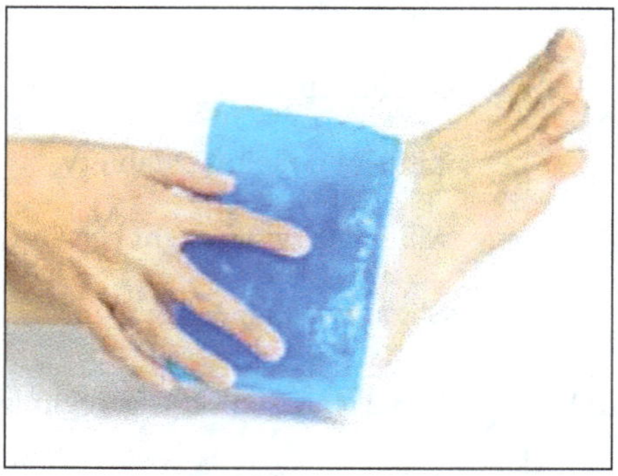

Treatment involves immediate first aid to reduce pain and swelling, rest to allow healing, followed by a rehabilitation program to restore full mobility, strength, and proprioception.

Self-help Treatment

- Apply the PRICE principles (protection, rest, ice, compression and elevation) as soon as possible after injury. It is important to rest the ankle to prevent further damage.
- Apply ice wrapped in a wet tea towel to prevent ice burns, or better still a cold therapy and compression wrap will reduce pain, inflammation, and swelling.
- Cold therapy can be applied for 10 mins every hour initially, reducing the frequency as symptoms improve. Elevating the ankle can also help reduce swelling by allowing tissue fluids to drain away.
- Wear an ankle brace or support to protect the injured ligaments and provide compression. Initially, a simple elastic compression sleeve or support is ideal, whilst later in the rehabilitation process, a stronger brace with additional lateral support at the side may help protect the ligaments.
- When pain allows, a full rehabilitation program of mobilizing, strengthening and finally functional or sports specific exercises should be performed.

What can a Professional Therapist do?

- A professional therapist can accurately diagnose your injury and give advice on treatment and rehabilitation.
- They may use electrotherapy, such as ultrasound to help relieve pain, relax the muscles and reduce swelling.
- Sports massage may be used to help reduce swelling in the acute stage and later cross friction massage directly to the ligament can help prevent scar tissue formation.

Sprained Ankle Taping

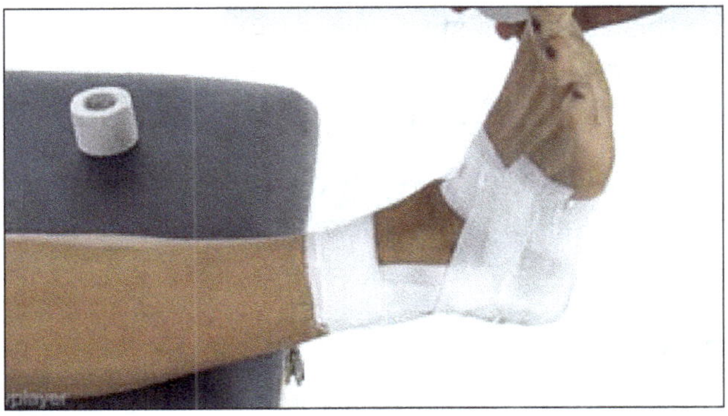

Taping for ankle sprains is used to both protect your injured ankle and improve confidence following injury. Tape can help support the damaged tissues in your ankle and activate the surrounding muscles. A professional therapist can tape your ankle, or you can try applying the tape at home by following the methods shown in our videos.

An expert will also be able to advise on rehabilitation exercises. Because they can assess the injury and where the damage has been done, they can recommend the best and most effective exercises for you to do. These exercises also involve strengthening the ankle and looking at any weaknesses that may have contributed to the injury. Performing these can help prevent any further injury in the future.

> "People often say they have 'weak' ankles but in most cases, they have ankles that are in fact "poor proprioceptively" and not weak at all. Proprioception is by far the most effective treatment for treating and is the secret to preventing re-injuries in ankle injuries."
>
> –Neal Reynolds, Sports Physiotherapist

Exercises for a Sprained Ankle

Strengthening, mobility and proprioceptive exercises are important in the rehabilitation of ankle sprains.

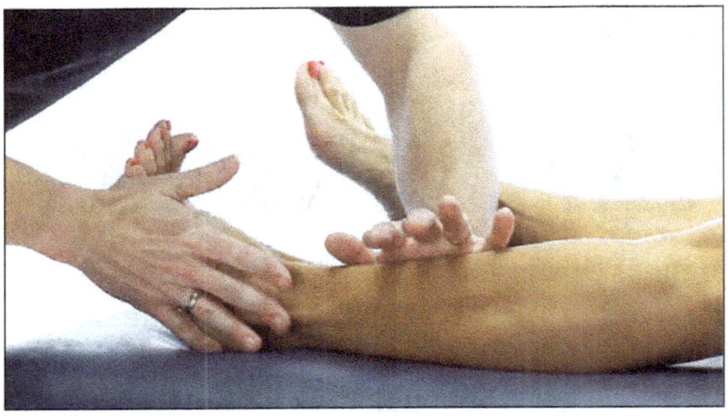

Stretching and Mobility Exercises

Mobility exercises for the ankle can start very early in the rehabilitation process from day 2 in mild to moderate sprains. As a sprain can make the joint stiff, performing mobility exercises and stretches will help maintain normal range of movement.

Sideways movements should be avoided early on so as not to put any stress at all on the injured ligaments. Later, when pain allows, exercises with lateral movements involving sideways motion can be done.

Strengthening Exercises

Ankle strengthening exercises can begin as soon as pain allows. Exercises that involve sideways movements should be avoided in the early stages to protect the healing ligaments. Isometric eversion and inversion exercises help to control the 'rolling' action of the ankle. This is especially helpful in preventing future injuries. A therapist or a friend can provide resistance, or you could use a wall.

Proprioceptive and Functional Exercises

One of the most important parts of ankle injury rehabilitation and in preventing re-injuries is proprioception. It is essential that proprioception exercises are included. These 'fire up' the muscles around the ankle joint to prevent injuries from reoccurring. Proprioception exercises include standing on one leg (which can be increased in difficulty by closing your eyes and standing on an unstable surface) to hopping (when pain allows).

Ankle Sprain Taping

Ankle Taping Figure of 8

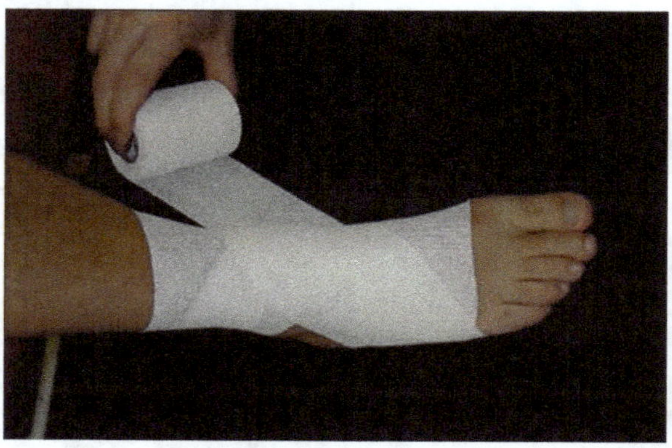

The figure of 8 strapping is the first and probably least supportive stage of ankle strapping. It aims to protect either the lateral ligaments on the outside or the deltoid ligaments on the inside of the ankle. Most ankle sprains will result in torn or stretched lateral ligaments on the outside of the ankle.

Equipment needed – Adhesive spray, underwrap, elastic adhesive bandage, and non-stretch zinc oxide tape. The underwrap is optional and used if someone is particularly hairy. Some athletes prefer to shave the leg to enable better contact and support from the tape rather than use underwrap. The adhesive is used to prevent the underwrap moving against the skin.

Some types of elastic tape can be torn by hand, others require scissors to cut them. The tearable tape is preferable for using pitch side because it can be applied more quickly.

Step 1 – Get the patient to hold their foot up, toes pointing upwards (dorsiflexion position). It is important that the patient keeps their foot in this position because if they relax in whilst the tape is being applied then it may become far too loose. Any strapping will gradually become loose once the patient begins to walk so it is important it is done properly to start with. It is also important not to apply the tape too tightly as once the patient walks around the foot may swell and blood flow will be restricted.

Step 2 – Apply adhesive spray to the leg and wrap the underwrap (if used) around the foot and ankle overlapping as you go.

Step 3 – Ensure the patient's foot is in the dorsiflexed position and starting on the inside of the ankle apply a support strip of elastic adhesive bandage up and across the inside of the ankle, then down under the foot to the outside of the ankle. Make sure the tape is not pulled too tightly as it passes underneath and up the outside of the heel.

Step 4 – Pass the tape across the front of the ankle, then around the back of the ankle (and Achilles) to make a figure of 8.

Step 5 – Pass the tape across the front of the ankle and down the inside and under the foot again the same as before, but slightly back towards the heel. The tape is then once more passed across the front of the ankle and behind the Achilles as before.

Step 6 – Then, instead of passing under the foot a third time, wrap around the ankle to cover the tape edges of previous passes, then down the inside, under the foot, up the outside and finish at the ankle.

If the taping has been done well there will be no creases in the tape, or gaps at the back of the heel as these can cause blisters.

Stirrups

An ankle strapping can have different stages or levels of support. Stage 1 demonstrated a figure of 8 technique which can be used on its own or applied before applying stage 2 stirrups.

Heel lock

The third stage of ankle strapping follows a figure of 8 first stage which is the least supportive followed by stirrup straps which protect the lateral ligaments. Any of these taping techniques can be used on their own as required of all together for maximum support.

Basketweave Ankle Strapping

This stage 4 of the ankle strapping technique called a basketweave technique. It is the most supportive of all of the ankle strapping techniques. It supports the lateral ligament complex on the outside and the deltoid ligament complex on the inside.

GROIN STRAIN

A groin strain is a tear of the adductor muscles on the inside of the thigh. A sudden sharp pain is felt which can range from a mild to very severe.

Groin Strain Symptoms and Diagnosis

The main symptom of a groin strain is sudden sharp pain on the inside of the thigh. It can be either in the belly of the muscle, or higher up where the tendon attaches to the pelvis. Often pain is felt when sprinting or changing direction quickly. The athlete may or may not be able to play on depending on how severe the injury is.

Although there is often swelling as a result of a groin strain, this is often not visible to the eye. Groin strains are graded 1, 2 or 3 depending on the extent of the injury.

- Grade 1

  A Grade 1 strain is a minor tear where less than 25% of fibers are damaged. You will most likely have discomfort in the groin area, but be able to walk with little or no pain. Often it is not possible to recall the exact point of injury as pain may only be noticeable after exercise. If you press into the muscle it may feel tight or tender. Stretching the groin muscles may also reproduce pain. Fast, explosive movements are mosts likely to trigger pain.

- Grade 2

  A Grade 2 injury is a moderate tear which involves damage to more than 25% of fibres. You will often know when the injury occurred from a sudden sharp pain in the groin during exercise. Bruising and swelling will develop over the next few days, but will not always be visible. Attempting to contract the muscle against resistance will be painful. This is easily tested by squeezing a ball between your knees. Pain will also be felt on stretching the groin muscles.

- Grade 3

  Grade 3 groin strains are the most serious. They involve either a complete (100%)

or almost complete rupture of the muscle. You will feel severe pain at the time of injury and be unable to continue. Contracting the groin muscles will be impossible from a combination of pain and weakness. Substantial swelling and bruising will usually develop around the inner thigh area and this may become visible within 24 to 48 hours.

Assessment Tests

A professional therapist will perform a full examination which includes a number of tests:

Range of motion – Testing the range of motion available at the hip joint or stretching the suspected injured muscles may reproduce symptoms. By identifying which movements are most painful, your therapist can deduce which muscles/tendons may be injured. Moving the leg out to the side (away from the body into abduction) stretches the groin muscles and can give an indication about flexibility. In a healthy athlete, both legs should be equal in terms of degree of stretch or flexibility.

Resisted Muscle Tests – These involve the therapist applying resistance as the patient takes the injured leg through a range of movement. Muscle tests should be done with your leg in different positions to isolate individual muscles. If you feel pain on any particular movement, this indicates the type and location of your injury.

Imaging – An Ultrasound scan or MRI may be used to confirm the diagnosis where available.

Causes and Anatomy

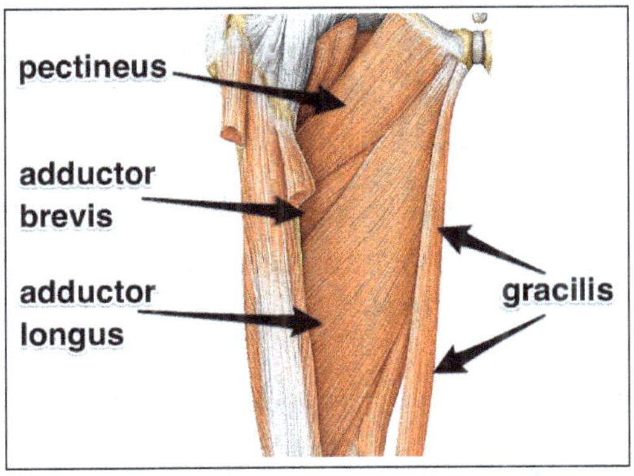

There are five groin (adductor) muscles. Three of them are called the 'short adductors' (pectineus, adductor brevis, and adductor longus). The other two are known as the 'long adductors' (gracilis and adductor Magnus).

Functions of Adductor Muscles

The main function of the adductor muscle group is to pull the leg back towards the midline. This movement called adduction. The adductor muscles also stabilize and control the pelvis during most activities including walking, running, sprinting, playing football, horse riding and hurdling. They are especially important in any sport which requires rapid changes in direction. The adductor muscles on one side keep the pelvis level while the adductor muscles on the opposite side are used to move the leg.

Cause of Groin Muscle Strains

Although muscle strains can occur randomly there are factors which can increase the likelihood of sustaining a groin strain. These include not warming up properly, having weak adductor muscles, tight adductor muscles, previous injury, lower back problems, and biomechanical factors.

Groin strains usually occur when sprinting or changing direction quickly or during rapid movements of the leg against resistance such as kicking a ball. Overstretching the muscle such as in martial arts high kicks can also cause a torn adductor muscle. There is likely to be damage to more than one structure in sudden onset or acute groin strains.

Groin Strain Treatment and Rehabilitation

Groin strain rehabilitation program is based on four strands or pathways of treatment (ice, heat, massage etc), stretching, strengthening and maintaining fitness. Each injury and each athlete is different and will start at a different point, and also progress at different rates.

Self-help Treatment

Apply the P.R.I.C.E principles (protection, rest, ice, compression, and elevation) as soon as possible after the injury and for the first 72 hours. A cold therapy and compression wrap will help stop internal bleeding, reduce pain and swelling speeding up the healing process. Wearing a groin support or groin strapping is also useful in the early stages in order to minimise pain and support the muscle while it heals. The use of groin supports and compression shorts is useful to protect and support the muscle when returning to training.

After the initial acute stage, a progressive stretching and strengthening exercise program is advised to ensure the muscle regains pre-injury levels of strength and flexibility and is, therefore, less prone to re-injury.

What can a Professional Therapist/Doctor do?

A professional therapist will assess the injury and make an accurate diagnosis. Electrotherapy modalities such as ultrasound may be used to aid the healing process. A doctor may prescribe NSAID medication such as Ibuprofen (do not take if you have asthma) to help with pain and swelling.

Groin Strain Strapping/Taping

Strapping the groin can aid healing by applying compression to the area immediately after injury. This is part of the PRICE principles of protection, rest, ice, compression, and elevation. It can also protect and support the muscles during rehabilitation and help prevent further damage to the injured muscle. A 7cm or 10cm elastic or elastic cohesive bandage and 2.5cm nonstretch zinc oxide tape is required to finish it off.

To strap the groin start on the inside of the thigh to be supported wrap once around the thigh applying tension across the front and upwards of the groin. Pass the bandage around the back of the waist and around to the front.

Then pass the bandage around the back of the thigh and around the groin once more applying tension to the front and upwards on the groin. Again, pass around the back and repeat this as required or until the bandage runs out.

Follow the same pattern with a roll of 2.5cm zinc oxide tape. Start on the inside of the groin, pass around the thigh applying tension as the tape comes around the groin and up the front of the thigh. Pass the tape around the back of the waist, across the front and then back around the thigh to the start.

Sports Massage

Sports massage may be beneficial once the acute stage has passed (after 72 hours) by releasing tension in the muscle and encouraging blood flow and nutrients. Caution is advised as massaging an injury too soon may increase the bleeding and may make the injury worse.

Groin Strain Exercises

After the initial acute stage of the injury has passed, a gradual rehabilitation program consisting of stretching and strengthening exercises should begin.

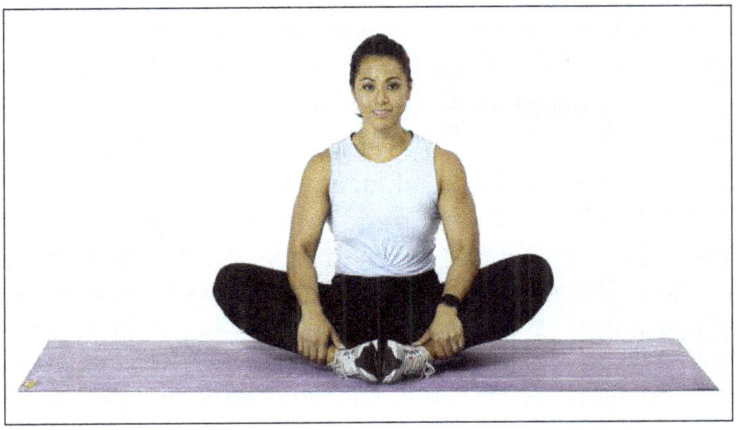

Stretching Exercises

Stretching should always be pain-free starting with gentle static stretches where the athlete eases into the stretch and hold for up to 30 seconds, repeating five times a day.

Long adductor stretch (legs straight), short adductor stretch (legs bent) and hip flexor stretching should be done ensuring all groin muscles are stretched.

These are progressed as the muscle heals to more dynamic exercises which involve movement or swinging of the leg. Do not start stretching too early as the healing of the muscle may be compromised (not before day 5 post-injury).

Strengthening exercises

The aim to gradually increase the load that is put through a muscle and can start as early as day 5 as long as they are low-level and pain-free. Isometric or static exercises are advised first and do not involve any movement of the muscle. For example, squeezing a medicine ball between the knees, or using a partner or therapist for resistance.

Eccentric exercises are more advanced exercises which focus on strengthening the muscle whilst it lengthens rather than shortens as all the previous exercises have done. A therapist or partner is needed to assist with this one. Dynamic exercises with a resistance band are performed as the muscle gains in strength.

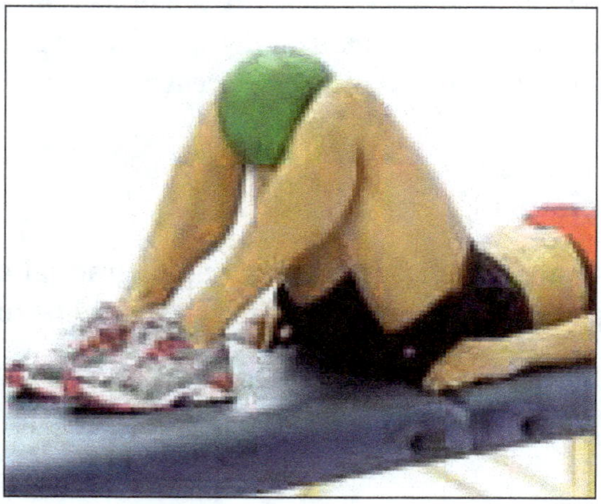

Straight leg raise and more advanced adduction exercises using gravity or resistance bands are done as pain allows leading on to even more dynamic and sports specific exercises which involve running, change of direction drills, hopping, and plyometric exercises. These bridge the gap between rehabilitation exercises and returning to full training and competition.

SHIN PAIN

Shin pain occurs most frequently in athletes involved in running, jumping, or high-impact sports. Shin pain can be caused by shin splints (also called medial tibial stress syndrome), a stress fracture of the tibia or fibula, or compartment syndrome. The most common source of shin pain in runners is shin splints.

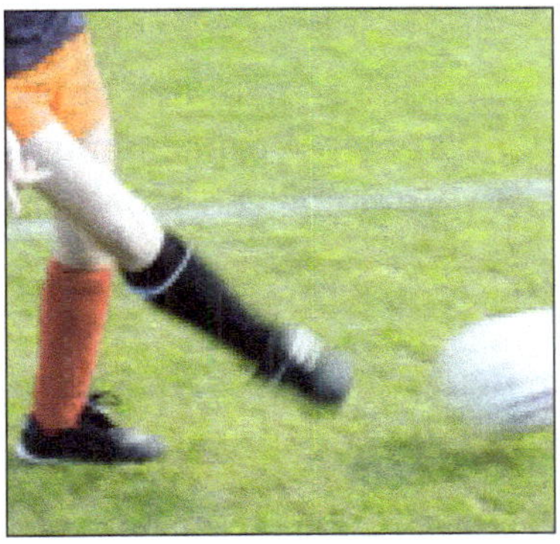

Symptoms

For all of the different causes of shin pain, athletes often complain first of pain, burning, or tightness along the shin. The following are symptoms of bone-related and musclerelated shin pain.

Symptoms of bone-related shin pain may include:

- Pain in a very focal area of the shin.
- Pain during and after running.
- Pain that gets worse over time.

Symptoms of muscle-related shin pain may include:

- Mild soreness.
- Tightness or pressure in shins with running.
- Pain only with running, relieved by rest.
- No pain when pushing on the bone.
- Numbness, tingling, or weakness in the foot.

Causes

Shin pain is generally the result of one or more of the following issues:

- Body mechanics refers to the way the body moves while in motion. Athletes may experience pain due to poor body mechanics. The way the body moves can be influenced by different factors. For example, how a runner runs may be affected by foot type, running style, and hip and core (abdominal and back) muscle strength.

- Too much exercise can become a problem if athletes increase too quickly. A helpful reminder is the "10% Rule": no more than a 10% increase in frequency, duration, or intensity of exercise per week.
- Bone density (bone strength). Softer bones break easier, so if there is a stress fracture that is not explained by poor mechanics or rapid increases in training, bone density might be the problem. The causes of low bone density include:
    - Genetics (it tends to run in families).
    - Not enough calcium in the diet (more than 1,300 mg/day is the recommended daily amount, equal to 3 to 4 servings of milk, yogurt, cheese, or other sources).
    - Irregular periods (no menstrual period for more than 6 months in a row), which causes low levels of the hormone estrogen.

Tests

Shin splints can be diagnosed by their characteristic symptoms and physical examination findings. A stress fracture is suspected when shin pain becomes more severe, more localized (in a focal area), or if there are risk factors for weaker bones such as the female athlete triad. X-rays may show a stress fracture if the problem has been present long enough to see a healing response (4–6 weeks). However, x-rays can appear normal even when a stress fracture is known to be present. In order to confirm the presence of a stress fracture, it may be necessary for magnetic resonance imaging (MRI).

Athletes with compartment syndromes will have normal x-rays and no evidence of bony abnormalities with bone scan or MRI. Compartment syndrome is confirmed by taking a pressure measurement through a needle inserted into the muscle both before and after exercise.

Treatment

A period of rest from running may be needed for the stress fracture or shin splints to heal. Although the athlete may be able to run with shin splints, continuing to do so may cause the shin splints to progress to a stress fracture. During rest, cross-training with nonimpact activities (such as using an elliptical machine, biking, swimming, and weights) can be done if the athlete is pain-free. Ice and acetaminophen are effective for pain, but nonsteroidal anti-inflammatory drugs (NSAIDs) such as ibuprofen or naproxen may actually slow the healing of some stress fractures. Other treatments like bone stimulators are controversial. In very rare cases rest is not enough for a fracture to heal, and surgery is needed.

Prevention

Shin splints and stress fractures can be reduced by allowing time to gradually build up to higher levels of impact activity (increase by no more than 10% per week). If an athlete has flat feet or high-arched feet, a proper shoe and/or shoe insert may be helpful. Since stress fractures in the shin usually start with shin splints, identifying and treating shin splints—before they progress—can prevent the development of stress fractures. Maintaining healthy bone through good diet (high in vitamin D and calcium), safe weight loss practices, and attention to any menstrual problems may also reduce the risk of stress fracture.

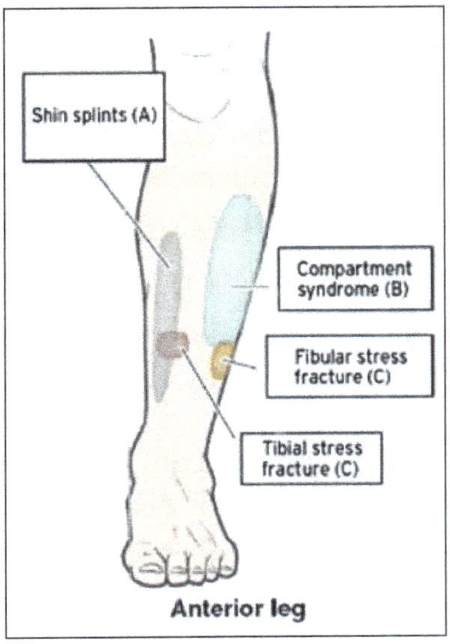

Compartment syndromes are more difficult to prevent. However, balancing low-impact conditioning with high-impact conditioning, selecting softer surfaces for running, and using a properly cushioned running shoe may help.

HAMSTRING INJURIES

Hamstring (HS) muscle injuries are the most common injury in sports. They are correlated to long rehabilitations and have a great tendency to recur. The HS consist of the long head of the biceps femoris, semitendinosus, and semimembranosus. The patient's clinical presentation depends on the characteristics of the lesion, which may vary from strain to avulsions of the proximal insertion. The most recognized risk factor is a previous injury. Magnetic resonance imaging is the method of choice for the injury diagnosis and classification. Many classification systems have been proposed; the current classifications aim to describe the injury and correlate it to the prognosis. The treatment is conservative, with the use of anti-inflammatory drugs in the acute phase followed by a muscle rehabilitation program. Proximal avulsions have shown better results with surgical repair. When the patient is pain free, shows recovery of strength and muscle flexibility, and can perform the sport's movements, he/she is able to return to play. Prevention programs based on eccentric strengthening of the muscles have been indicated both to prevent the initial injury as well as preventing recurrence.

Historically, hamstring (HS) injuries are described as frustrating for athletes as they are correlated with a long rehabilitation time; they have a tendency to recur and return to sport is unpredictable.

Not all injuries are similar. They range from mild muscle damage to complete tear of muscle fibers. Furthermore, as with the characteristics of the lesions, rehabilitation time is also variable.

HS injuries are the most common in sports. They are the most frequently reported injuries in soccer, accounting for 37% of the muscular injuries observed in that sport, which is the most popular in the world, with over 275 million practitioners.

Injury incidence is estimated at 3–4.1/1000 h of competition and 0.4–0.5/1000 h of training. A mean increase of 4% per year has been reported; the rate of injuries occurring in training sessions has increased more than that of those occurring during competitive activities. After the injury, runners need 16 weeks, on average, to return to sport without restrictions, while dancers can take up to 50 weeks. In professional soccer, the athlete remains, on average, 14 days away from competitive activities. HS injury is the main cause of injury absence.

In addition to soccer, injuries are common in sports such as football, Australian football, track and field, and water skiing. The most common trauma mechanism is indirect trauma; injuries tend to occur during non-contact activities, and running is the primary activity. Sports that require ballistic movements of the lower limb, such as skiing, dancing, and skating, are associated with proximal avulsion of the HS tendons.

The myotendinous junction (MTJ) is the most vulnerable part of the muscle, tendon, and bone junction; the more proximal the injury, the longer the return to sport activity.

Of all muscle injuries, those of HS have one of the highest recurrence rates, which is estimated to range between 12% and 33%. Recurrence is the most common complication of HS lesions.

Anatomy

The HS muscle group consists of the semitendinosus (ST), semimembranosus (SM), and the long head of the biceps femoris (LHBF). These three muscles originate in the ischial tuberosity (IT) as a common tendon, passing through the hip and knee joints; they are biarticular muscles and are innervated by the tibial portion of the sciatic nerve. In the posterior region of the thigh, the short head of the biceps femoris (SHBF), which originates in the posterolateral region of the femur in the linea aspera and in the supracondylar ridge, is added to the HS group. Thus, the SHBF is a monoarticular muscle innervated by the common fibular nerve

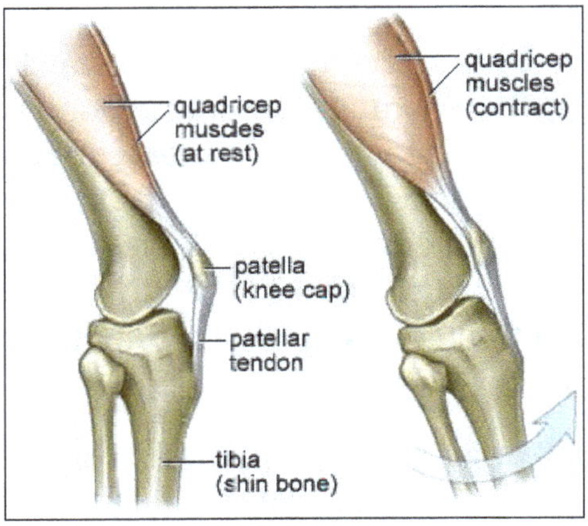

Schematic drawing of the hamstrings.

In an anatomical study of the HS, Van der Made et al. described that the HS is divided into two portions, upper and lower. The upper portion is subdivided into two facets. The lateral facet is the origin of SM, whereas the medial facet is the origin of the ST and LHBF, which also has origins in the sacrotuberal ligament.

The ST and SM extend to the posteromedial region of the thigh, with insertions in the pes anserinus and the posteromedial corner of the knee and tibia, respectively. In an agonistic pattern, these muscles act in knee flexion and medial rotation, as well as in hip extension; laterally, the LHBF acts in an isolated manner proximally, extending the hip and posterior stabilizing the pelvis. The distal tendon that is inserted in the head of the fibula is formed distally, after the addition of the SHBF fibers, which flex the knee with the thigh in extension.

To date, no hypothesis has been able to correlate injury patterns with the anatomical structure based solely on the length of the muscle, tendon, or MTJ. It is thought that the muscular architecture, due to the proximal and distal orientations of the tendons, leads to a resulting force that is misaligned with the muscular fibers, predisposing to injury. A tendinous structure in the ST divides it into two parts. This raphe may play a role in protecting against gross injuries of this muscle.

Clinical Picture

Clinical presentation of the patient depends on the characteristics of the lesion, which can range from stretching of the muscle fibers to tendon rupture. Nonetheless, regardless of strains or ruptures, proximal lesions are much more common than distal lesions. The LHBF is the most frequently injured muscle and, despite the lack of consensus, the SM is considered to be the second most affected muscle.

Askling et al. proposed two types of acute injuries. First type occurs during sprinting, and affects the LHBF. The second type is associated with excessive HS stretching in movements such as kicking in soccer or tackling in football, and most often affects the SM.

Eccentric contraction is the muscular action in which the fibers are elongated as a result of an external force, and at the same time contract to decelerate the movement. In indirect trauma, the maximum eccentric contraction period appears to present the greatest risk for muscle injury; the most common injury site is the MTJ, since it bears the greatest eccentric loads. Direct trauma is another mechanism of injury, especially in sports with body contact. It is less frequent and is mainly associated with lesions of the muscular bellies. In the HS, delayed onset muscle soreness is induced by eccentric contraction, representing another common sports-related condition.

Proximal avulsion of the HS origin corresponds to 12% of these lesions. It is estimated that 9% of these are complete avulsions, which is considered to be the most serious. The typical mechanism of proximal avulsion is eccentric contraction of the HS, as a result of sudden hip hyperflexion, with the knee in extension. This movement is most commonly observed in water skiing.

Clinically, patient presents with a sudden pain in the posterior region of the thigh. The report of an audible click and the inability to continue with physical activity is common. Antalgic gait develops to minimize mobilization of the involved muscle mass and decrease hip extension and knee flexion. In the acute phase, the most common clinical signs are hematoma or ecchymosis in the posterior region of the thigh, painful palpation of the IT region, and muscle weakness. Usually, hematoma volume is correlated with lesion severity, but its absence cannot be confused with a minor lesion, since this sign may be late even in the most severe lesions.

HS strength can be tested through knee flexion and hip extension against resistance. A bilateral comparison is indicated to identify the alterations. The "taking off the shoe" clinical test is also described as a means of assessing the HS. The patient is asked to remove the shoe ipsilateral to the injury in the standing position, with the help of the contralateral foot. By leveraging the back of the foot on the contralateral limb, the patient will flex the knee and trigger pain or demonstrate the weakness of the affected muscles.

In proximal avulsion, a local gap may be palpable, but sometimes it can be masked by the hematoma. Discomfort in sitting may be reported; palpation helps to identify the location and which muscles are injured. Complete rupture is defined as the rupture of the three HS tendons (BF, ST, and SM). The rope sign has been proposed to differentiate between partial and complete tendon avulsion. A positive test is characterized by the absence of palpable tension in the distal part of the HS with the patient in the prone position, with the knee flexed to 90°. Avulsion can also be evaluated in cases of knee flexion against resistance, when the avulsed muscle mass retracts distally.

Neurological clinical examination should always be performed in case of HS injury. Due to local proximity, muscle injuries may be correlated with neurological lesions, which may manifest with paresthesia or motor alterations. In the chronic phases of the lesions, sciatica symptoms may arise.

In the acute phase, the pain picture greatly impacts the clinical evaluation of the patient. After 48 h, the acute limitation of pain is expected to have decreased, and the result of the physical examination may be more relevant both for diagnosis and for prognosis. Therefore, specific evaluation is indicated within two days after the injury.

Differential diagnoses range from HS apophysitis, piriformis syndrome, tendinopathies, and bursitis to radiculopathies. Therefore, clinical history, patient's complaint, and physical examination are crucial for the correct diagnosis.

Risk Factors

Many studies have sought to identify the risk factors for HS injury. The ability to recognize the athletes with predisposition and the situations that can lead to injury is paramount for prevention, in order to avoid long periods of rehabilitation and injury leave.

Among the risk factors, the specific characteristics of the muscles play an important role. HS muscle imbalance is defined by the difference in muscle strength when compared with the contralateral side, or an alteration in the ratio of HS strength to ipsilateral quadriceps strength. The risk of injury is higher when the strength deficit between the HS is >10–15%, or when the strength ratio between the HS and the quadriceps is <0.6. However, these values may vary according to each athlete and sport.

The sporting motion is also a predisposing factor of injury. Athletes who anteriorly tilt the pelvis at the moment of acceleration during the stride increase the tension on the HS. Furthermore, iliopsoas shortening and imbalance of the abdominal and lumbar musculature may also promote pelvic anteversion, placing the HS at a mechanical disadvantage by increasing muscle tension at the end of the swing phase of the gait cycle.

Extrinsic factors can also influence the probability of injury. Injuries are more common during competitions than training; short pre-seasons are also correlated with a greater chance of injury. Athletes who have to run due to their positions are at greater risk of injury. In soccer, injuries on the dominant side are more serious, as they are correlated with the kicking movement.

Previous HS injury is the risk factor most commonly correlated with new lesions. Injury recurrence after returning to sport remains the main complication of this pathology. Recurrence is more common when the lesion involves the LHBF. Van Beijsterveldt et al. conducted a systematic review of 11 prospective studies involving 1775 male soccer players with 334 HS injuries. These authors observed that prior HS lesion was significantly correlated with risk for a new lesion. HS injury recurrence rates are reported to range from 14% to 63% within two years after the initial injury.

Pruna et al. hypothesized that the genetic profile could explain why some elite soccer players are more predisposed to injuries than others, as well as the reason for the marked time variation in the rehabilitation of injuries.

Regarding proximal HS avulsions, complete ruptures tend to occur in patients with previous local tendinopathy.

Imaging Tests

Imaging tests confirm the diagnosis and provide information for therapeutic decision-making.

As a first modality, the radiographic study is indicated for ruling out HS avulsion fractures, especially in skeletally immature patients.

Ultrasonography (US) has the advantage of being affordable and inexpensive; however, it is operator-dependent. The examination should be performed between the second and seventh days after the trauma; that injury can be detected through visualization of the hematoma and the discontinuity of the fibers. It is also possible to measure the length, width, depth, and cross-sectional area of the muscle injury. In proximal cases, this method has greater limitations to measure this lesion.

Magnetic resonance imaging (MRI) is the modality of choice for identifying and describing lesions, especially those of proximal location. It precisely defines the site of injury, its severity and extension, the involved tendons, and the retraction of muscle mass.

There is still no consensus on the optimal moment for MRI assessment. Some authors advocate that the test should be performed between 24 h and 48 h after trauma, while others advocate that this interval should be between 48 h and 72 h. The signs of the lesion are mainly recognized in T2-weighted images with fat suppression or in short-tau inversion recovery (STIR); they are more apparent from 24 h up to five days after trauma.

Although MRI is the gold standard exam, 13% of HS lesions in professional soccer players may not be identified by MRI. The reason for this is still unknown. One hypothesis is that these are small lesions that are not detectable, another is that the symptoms may be caused by other pathologies, such as low back pain or neurological changes.

For follow-up of the injuries, MRI is more sensitive than US. The images would be useful in more severe cases and in the assessment of progression and rehabilitation, aiding in the decision of return to sport in elite athletes. In 34–94% of cases, signs of HS injury are still visible after six weeks.

Classification

Classification systems are useful for physicians, athletes, and their coaches, as they guide treatment and prognosis. A wide variety of classifications based on clinical signs and alterations in US and MRI imaging tests has been proposed. However, due to the complexity and heterogeneity of muscle injuries, there is still no widely accepted classification system.

In clinical practice, a three-degree system is the most commonly used, classifying the injury as minor, moderate, or complete muscle tear. Variations correlated with imaging tests have also been described.

Peetrons grouped lesions into grades, according to the alterations observed in the US. Grade i includes lesions that do not present alteration in the muscular architecture, but have signs of edema around the muscle. Grade ii includes partial ruptures, and Grade III injuries present complete muscle or tendon tear.

Recently, new classification systems have been developed; these systems aim to be more comprehensive and to standardize the terminology of muscle injury, as well as to provide each degree of injury with a prognosis, which does not occur in the three-degree classification.

It proposes a classification system for muscle injury based on MRI images. Injuries are graded from 0 to 4; in grades 1 to 4, an additional suffix describes the location of the lesion (a, for myofascial lesions; b, for musculotendinous lesions; and c, for intra-tendinous lesions).

Table: British athletics muscle injury classification.

Grade	Description	MRI
Grade 0		
0a	Focal neuromuscular pain	Normal.
0b	Generalized muscle soreness after exercise	Normal or increased signal in one or more muscles.
Grade 1		
1a	Minor myofascial injury	Increased signal from the fascia involving <10% of the muscle belly, and craniocaudal length <5 cm.
1b	Minor myotendinous injury	Signal increase <10% of the transverse section of muscle in the myotendinous area and craniocaudal length <5 cm.
Grade 2		
2a	Moderate myofascial injury	Increased signal from the fascia extending to the muscle, lesion cross-sectional area of 10% and 50%, craniocaudal length >5 and <15 cm, structural fiber disruption <5 cm.
2b	Moderate myotendinous injury	Increased signal in the myotendinous region, lesion cross-sectional area ranging from 10% and 50%, craniocaudal length >5 and <15 cm, structural fiber disruption <5 cm.
2c	Moderate intratendinous injury	Increased signal in the tendon, with longitudinal length <5 cm and <50% of the cross-sectional area of the tendon is involved. No loss of tendon tension or discontinuity are observed.
Grade 3		
3a	Extensive myofascial injury	Increased signal from the fascia extending to the muscle, lesion cross-sectional area >50%, craniocaudal length >15 cm, structural fiber disruption > 5 cm.
3b	Extensive myotendinous injury	Increased signal with lesion cross-sectional area >50%, craniocaudal length >15 cm, and structural fiber disruption > 5 cm.

3c	Extensive intratendinous injury	Increased signal in the tendon, with longitudinal length >5 cm and >50% of the cross-sectional area of the tendon is involved. Loss of tendon tension may be observed, but there is no apparent discontinuity.
Grade 4		
4	Complete muscle injury	Complete muscle discontinuity with retraction.
4c	Complete tendon injury	Complete discontinuation of tendon with retraction.

Grade 0 injuries present no alteration on MRI. This grade represents focal neuromuscular pain and generalized muscle pain caused by exercise. Grade 1 injuries are minor muscle injuries in which the athlete experiences pain during or after the activity. Range of motion (ROM) is normal and the strength is preserved. In Grade 2 injuries, moderate muscle damage is observed. The athlete presents pain during the activity and must interrupt it. The ROM of the affected limb is limited due to pain, and muscle weakness is usually detected upon clinical examination. In Grade 3, muscle injuries are extensive. The athlete usually suffers an abrupt pain, and may fall. Even after 24 h, ROM is usually reduced and the pain picture persists. There is an obvious muscle contractility weakness. Finally, Grade 4 represents complete muscle or tendon tear. The athlete presents sudden pain and activity limitation. A palpable gap can be perceived. Normally, the contraction is less painful than that observed in Grade 3 injuries.

The clinical application of the British Athletics Muscle Injury Classification was demonstrated by Pollock et al. in a study that assessed 65 HS lesions in 44 track and field athletes. The higher the grade of the lesion, the longer the time of rehabilitation and the higher the rate of relapse. Cases with tendon involvement (type C) were more susceptible to relapse and had a longer rehabilitation time.

In below table shows, distinguishes between two main groups of muscle injuries: Injury by direct or indirect trauma. Within the group of injuries due to indirect trauma, the classification brings the concept of functional and structural lesions. Functional muscle injuries present alterations without macroscopic evidence of fiber tear. These lesions have multifactorial causes and are grouped into subgroups that reflect their clinical origin, such as overload or neuromuscular disorders. Structural muscle injuries are those whose MRI study presents macroscopic evidence of fiber tear, i.e., structural damage. They are usually located in the MTJ, as these areas have biomechanical weak points.

Table: Munich classification.

Type of injury		Definition	Symptoms	MRI
Direct		Contusion: blunt trauma from external factor, with intact muscle tissue		Hematoma
		Laceration: blunt trauma from an external factor with muscular rupture		Hematoma

Indirect	Functional	Type 1: overload-related muscle disorder		
		1A: fatigue-induced muscle disorder	Muscle stiffness	Negative
		1B: delayed onset muscle soreness	Acute inflammatory pain	Negative or isolated edema
		Type 2: muscle disorder of neuromuscular origin		
		2A: spine-related neuromuscular muscle disorder	Increased muscle tone due to neurological disorder	Negative or isolated edema
		2B: muscle-related neuromuscular muscle disorder	Increased muscle tone due to altered neuromuscular control	Negative or isolated edema
	Structural	Type 3: Partial muscle tear		
		3A: minor partial muscle tear: tear involving a small area of the maximal muscle diameter		Fiber rupture
		3B: moderate partial muscle tear: tear involving moderate area of maximum muscle diameter		Retraction and hematoma
		Type 4: (sub)total muscle tear with avulsion:		
		Involvement of the entire muscle diameter, muscle defect		Complete discontinuation of fibers

Ekstrand et al. prospectively analyzed 31 professional men's soccer teams during the 2011/2012 season, in accordance with the Munich classification. A total of 393 thigh muscle injures were recorded; two-thirds of them were classified as structural and had a rehabilitation time (in which the athlete was unable to complete) that was significantly higher than that observed in functional injuries. Within structural lesions, significant differences were also observed in the subgroups (minor, moderate, and complete injury); the greater the severity, the longer the time to return to sport. In the present study, no significant differences were observed outcomes of anterior or posterior thigh muscle injuries.

Treatment

Most HS lesions are muscle strains or partial lesions at the MTJ level that can be conservatively managed and generally result in full recovery.

In the initial phase, treatment aims to minimize intramuscular bleeding and control inflammatory response. Analgesia, rest, ice packs, muscle compression, and limb elevation are used. However, clinical evidence to support the use of these treatment modalities is still limited. The best treatment for HS injuries is yet to be identified.

A greater emphasis on pain reduction in the first days after injury is necessary, because it reduces the neuromuscular inhibition associated with pain. Moreover, unnecessary immobilization should be avoided, as it leads to muscle atrophy. With early mobilization through stretching and strengthening exercises, a stable and functional healing is expected.

The inflammatory reaction, triggered in response to injury, is responsible for the onset of tissue repair. However, as a result of the enzymes released after cell lesion, the process also causes tissue degradation, which, together with local ischemia resulting from trauma to the blood supply, increases the muscle injury by involving the adjacent tissue and increasing inflammatory symptoms, such as pain and edema. Anti-inflammatory medication is indicated to modulate the inflammatory response and to control pain, allowing early initiation of rehabilitation. Non-steroidal anti-inflammatory drugs are the most used, and are indicated until the first 48–72 h of the lesion, to avoid interfering with tissue repair. After this phase, analgesics are used for antalgic management.

Corticosteroids can also be used for inflammation control, both orally and intramuscularly. Intralesion administration, which may be guided by US, is indicated when the acute condition does not present pain improvement and the patient has difficulty to perform the rehabilitation program. However, local use of corticosteroids may have deleterious effects on muscle tissue, because they act on collagen bonds and decrease tissue healing.

Treatment of Proximal Avulsions

HS lesions due to proximal tendon avulsion may lead to significant sequelae, such as strength deficit and inability to return to sports practice at the pre-injury level. Surgical repair of the local anatomy is indicated to avoid such complications, especially in athletes or physically active patients. In most surgical techniques described, the repair is performed using anchors and non-absorbable suture.

Hofmann et al. assessed the outcome of conservative treatment for complete proximal avulsions of the HS. A total of 30% of the patients were unable to return to the pre-injury level of sports activity, and almost half of them regretted not having undergone surgical treatment.

Barnett et al. reported that good-to-excellent results can be expected in most patients after surgical reinsertion of proximal avulsion of the HS. These authors also reported a high percentage of patients who returned to their pre-injury level; the vast majority of patients was satisfied with surgery and would opt for the same treatment again.

In general, conservative therapy is indicated for single-tendon acute proximal tendon avulsions or multiple tendon lesions with less than 2 cm of retraction. Asymptomatic chronic lesions, despite dislocation, are also treated conservatively.

Surgical treatment is the best option for ischial apophysis avulsions in skeletally immature patients, avulsions with the HS bone fragment, and proximal avulsions of the entire HS complex.

The surgery is also indicated for patients with active avulsions in one or two tendons and retraction greater than 2 cm. In recreational athletes or inactive patients, surgery is indicated only when the avulsion is symptomatic. Surgery may also be indicated in tendon injuries when avulsion is symptomatic, particularly in athletes or highly active patients. Theoretically, an LHBF avulsion may require surgical repair, since no other muscle acts as an agonist, unlike the ST and MS, which act synergistically.

When the diagnosis of proximal avulsion is confirmed, the possibility of surgical treatment should be addressed as early as possible, in order to repair the lesion during the acute phase. The consensus indicates that reinsertion should ideally be performed within two weeks of injury. Early repair minimizes muscle atrophy and shortening, facilitates rehabilitation (by making it more predictable), and avoids surgical difficulties and complications, such as adhesions between the avulsed tissue and the sciatic nerve, which form around the end of the second week. In addition to sciatic nerve involvement, the posterior femoral cutaneous nerve and lower gluteal nerve can also be involved, causing dysesthesia and weakness of the hip extensors.

Injuries that are not surgically treated may evolve with neuralgia and sciatica. Surgical repair is also indicated in these chronic cases and in lesions that, despite conservative treatment, persist with debilitating pain and weakness. However, it is worth emphasizing that the neurological symptoms may persist after the surgical procedure.

Platelet-rich Plasma

Myogeny is not restricted to prenatal development; it also occurs in muscle regeneration after injury. Several growth factors have been suggested as regulators of this process. Platelets are known for their role in hemostasis, but they also mediate tissue injury repair, due to their ability to release growth factors, which lead to the stimulation of angiogenesis (responsible for neovascularization) and increased metabolic activity, with tendon and muscle tissue proliferation.

The indication for the use of platelet-rich plasma (PRP) is based on the concept that the growth factors released by platelets would increase the natural healing process, especially in tissues with low potential for cure; this claim is supported by many in vitro studies. Because of the potential to enhance the tissue repair process, PRP has been investigated as part of the therapeutic arsenal for many lesions, including those of the HS.

Hamid et al. studied patients with acute HS injuries classified as partial ruptures. They were randomly allocated for treatment with autologous PRP combined with a rehabilitation program, or for rehabilitation program alone. The primary outcome of the study was the time to return to sports. The authors also assessed level of pain and interference of pain over time. That study demonstrated that a single injection of 3 mL of autologous PRP combined with a rehabilitation program was significantly more effective in reducing pain severity, allowing a shorter time to return to sport after an acute HS injury.

Rossi et al. also described a study in which a single application of autologous PRP associated with a rehabilitation program was compared with rehabilitation program alone in partial HS lesions; these authors observed a significantly decrease in time to return to sport in the combined treatment. At two years of follow-up, no differences were observed between groups regarding recurrence rate.

In a study of 25 HS injuries in professional soccer players, Zanon et al.32 demonstrated that the use of PRP was safe; the authors did not report a decrease in recovery time, but did show a smaller scar and improved tissue repair in the MRI control images.

Reurink et al., in a randomized, multicenter, double-blinded study with 80 recreational athletes with HS lesions, did not observe statistically or clinically significant results to justify the use of PRP.

In addition to the isolated use of PRP, its associations have also been studied. In an animal model, Terada et al. demonstrated that PRP combined with the use of losartan promoted an improvement in skeletal muscle healing after contusion by increasing revascularization rate and muscle regeneration, as well as by inhibiting the development of fibrosis. Losartan has an antifibrotic action, and it is also a widely used antihypertensive. Its association with PRP would stimulate angiogenesis and inhibit the development of fibrosis.

Despite the various studies, there is still insufficient evidence to indicate the use of PRP in acute muscle injury. Due to the increase in popularity, its real effectiveness has been increasingly debated, especially regarding the process of muscle injury rehabilitation in physically active patients and in athletes, thus it represents an important area of research.

Current literature shows promising pre-clinical outcomes, but clinical findings are contradictory. A detailed analysis is hampered by the lack of standardization of study protocols, PRP preparation techniques, and outcome measures.

High quality studies are critical to confirm these preliminary results and provide scientific evidence to indicate the use of PRP. Further research is needed to standardize PRP preparation, administration regimens (including the volume to be applied), treatment duration and frequency, and application method (blind or guided by US).

Rehabilitation

The rehabilitation process is based on muscle stretching and strengthening programs, since tissue healing involves muscle regeneration and fibrosis formation. Early mobility minimizes disorganized healing of the fibers and, therefore, lesion recurrence.

Prognostic factors related to a long rehabilitation period include muscle injury observed on MRI, extensive lesion demonstrated on MRI, recurrent HS lesions, and indirect injury as the trauma mechanism.

The functional rehabilitation of HS lesions should be individualized to the needs of each patient; the overall goals are to restore pre-injury muscle strength and flexibility, as well as to relieve pain. Muscle strengthening is both a rehabilitation and prevention factor.

The process begins with concentric strengthening, which leads to clinical improvement; open kinetic chain exercises are used progressively to initiate eccentric strengthening. Eccentric strengthening exercises are more effective than concentric exercises, and should be performed with the muscle in a stretched, as they help to restore muscle length after injury.

Return to Sports Practice

Return to sports is the desired outcome after HS injuries. Isolated lesions of the LHBF involving <50% of the cross-sectional area and minimum perimuscular edema are correlated with a rapid return to sport, usually within seven days. Delayed return, after over two or three weeks, is correlated with lesions in multiple muscles, MTJ lesions, lesions involving the SHBF, lesions with a cross-sectional area greater than 75%, presence of retraction, and lesions with circumferential muscle edema. A delay in the recovery process is also associated with primary injury and indirect injury as the trauma mechanism.

The criteria for sports return are: absence of pain, ability to make the respective sporting movements without hesitation, recovery of strength and stretching of the involved muscle group, and the athlete's own confidence for returning to physical activity. The assessment of muscle strength can be determined by the isokinetic test. Restoration of limb strength compared to contralateral side (between 90% and 95%) and HS to quadriceps strength ratio between 50% and 60% are desirable.

Most HS relapses occur at the same site as the primary lesions, early after the return to sport; these new lesions are radiologically more severe. Specific exercise programs focused on preventing new injuries are highly recommended after returning to sports.

Prevention

Given the major complications of HS injuries, especially in athletes, prevention is still better than treatment and rehabilitation process, especially considering the threat of recurrence. Several studies have aimed to identify patterns that predict injury, in order to avoid or correct these situations.

Duhig et al., who assessed soccer players and their sprints using GPS devices, observed that athletes who developed HS injury traveled a greater distance than their two-year average for high-speed sprinting (>24 km/h) in the four weeks prior to the injury.

Van Dyk et al. do not recommend the isokinetic test to determine the association between strength differences and HS injury, as they were unable to determine the factors that would identify soccer players at risk for injury in a study on the relationship between the eccentric HS strength and concentric quadriceps strength in the isokinetic evaluation of 614 players over four seasons.

However, Dauty et al. studied all soccer players in the major French league between the 2001/02 and 2011/12 seasons by isokinetic testing. According to those authors, it is possible to predict the occurrence of HS injury based on the results of the test conducted at the beginning of the season.

Schache et al. reported that the asymmetric measures on isokinetic tests of maximal voluntary contractions of the HS muscles may be a useful clinical test to identify susceptibility to injury. In the case report of an elite Australian football player, the HS isokinetic test demonstrated that, over four weeks, the asymmetry between the maximum voluntary contraction was minimal (<1.2%); however, five days prior to the injury, the side that would be affected presented a reduction in the maximum voluntary contraction force of 10.9%.

Despite the discrepancy between the different results of the studies, with variant methodologies, muscle strengthening is considered to be the main prevention factor. Regarding muscle stretching, little has been shown about its prophylactic function. However, the most enduring clinical sign after HS injury is the reduction of muscle elongation; therefore, stretching is especially useful for rehabilitating the primary lesion and preventing relapse. HS stretching with the pelvis in anterior inclination has been shown to be more effective than the standard stretches.

Regarding muscle strengthening, Mendiguchia et al. reported that seven weeks of neuromuscular training focusing on the HS, combined with soccer training, was more effective than isolated training effective in improving concentric contraction force, specifically HS eccentric strength. This result ensures that the program maintains the athlete's performance and helps prevent HS injuries.

Porter and Rushton conducted a systematic review of the effectiveness of eccentric strengthening exercises in the prevention of HS injuries in male professional soccer athletes. Those authors concluded that, although sufficient evidence is still lacking, there is scientific support in the literature for the indication of this prevention modality.

In summary, many authors agree that an exercise program for eccentric HS strengthening may reduce the incidence of injury. The effectiveness of those programs can be explained by the fact that the injury typically occurs when the HS muscles act on the deceleration of knee extension through an eccentric contraction in the final swing phase during the stride, when they are elongated by hip flexion and knee extension. The force required for the deceleration is proportional to the speed and force applied in the sprint.

Nordic flexion is considered to be one of the most effective exercises in eccentric HS strengthening; it has been used with good results in professional soccer teams and amateur athletes. The exercise begins with the athlete kneeling with the thighs and trunk aligned, at a right angle to the legs. A training partner helps hold the feet and legs on the ground. The athlete initiates the activity by tilting the trunk toward the floor as slowly as possible, in order to increase the muscular load during the eccentric phase. When the trunk approaches the ground, the upper limbs are used to prevent the fall and push the athlete's back, minimizing the loading during the concentric phase.

Bourne et al. assessed the Nordic flexion through functional MR images and found that the HS that had suffered injury muscle were less activated than the contralateral side. They also showed that the ST is the most significantly activated muscle. Regarding the analysis by electromyography, the same group, in a different study,44 observed that, although not selective for LHBF, Nordic flexion presented the highest levels of activation in the eccentric contraction of this muscle when compared with the other exercises assessed in their study. Those authors concluded that the HS muscles are activated differently during hip or knee-based exercises. Thus, exercises based on hip extension are more selective in lateral activation, whereas those with knee flexion preferentially engage the medial musculature.

Laboratory parameters can also be used to prevent injury. Classically, creatine phosphokinase and lactate dehydrogenase are used as biochemical markers. Serum levels depend on age, gender, ethnicity, muscle mass, physical activity, and even weather conditions. These parameters should not be used for the diagnosis or prognosis of lesions, due to their low sensitivity and specificity. However, an increase in these parameters indicates an incomplete recovery from the muscular overload when compared with the athlete's baseline measurements. Special attention should be given to correcting factors that may predispose to injury.

KNEE INJURY

Anatomy of the Knee

While there are four bones that come together at the knee, only the femur (thighbone) and the tibia (shinbone) form the joint itself. The head of the fibula (strut bone on the outside of the leg) provides some stability, and the patella (kneecap) helps with joint and muscle function. Movement and weight-bearing occur where the ends of the femur called the femoral condyles match up with the top flat surfaces of the tibia (tibial plateaus).

There are two major muscle groups that are balanced and allow movement of the knee joint. When the quadriceps muscles on the front of the thigh contract, the knee extends or straightens. The hamstring muscles on the back of the thigh flex or bend the knee when they contract. The muscles cross the knee joint and are attached to the tibia by tendons. The quadriceps tendon is special, in that it contains the patella within its fibers. The patella allows the quadriceps muscle/tendon unit to work more efficiently. The quadriceps tendon is renamed the patellar tendon from the kneecap to its attachment in the tibia.

The stability of the knee joint is maintained by four ligaments, thick bands of tissue that stabilize the joint. The medial collateral ligament (MCL) and lateral collateral ligament (LCL) are on the sides of the knee and prevent the joint from sliding sideways. The anterior cruciate ligament (ACL) and posterior cruciate ligament (PCL) form an

"X" on the inside of the knee and prevent the knee from sliding back and forth. These limitations on knee movement allow the knee to concentrate the forces of the muscles on flexion and extension.

Inside the knee, there are two shock-absorbing pieces of cartilage called menisci (singular meniscus) that sit on the top surface of the tibia. The menisci allow the femoral condyle to move on the tibial surface without friction, preventing the bones from rubbing on each other. Without this cartilage covering, the friction of bone on bone would cause inflammation, or arthritis.

Bursas surround the knee joint and are fluid-filled sacs that cushion the knee during its range of motion. In the front of the knee, there is a bursa between the skin and the kneecap called the prepatellar bursa and another above the kneecap called the suprapatellar bursa (supra=above).

Each part of the anatomy needs to function properly for the knee to work. Acute injury or trauma as well as chronic overuse may cause inflammation and its accompanying symptoms of pain, swelling, redness, and warmth.

Types and Causes of Knee Injuries

While direct blows to the knee will occur, the knee is more susceptible to twisting or stretching injuries (hyperflexed/hyperextended), taking the joint through a greater range of motion than it was meant to tolerate.

If the knee is stressed from a specific direction, then the ligament trying to hold it in place against that force can stretch or tear. These injuries are called sprains. Sprains are graded as first, second, or third degree based upon how much damage has occurred. Grade-one sprains stretch the ligament but don't tear the fibers; grade-two sprains partially tear the fibers, but the ligament remains intact; and grade-three tears completely disrupt the ligament.

Twisting injuries to the knee put stress on the cartilage or meniscus and can pinch them between the tibial surface and the edges of the femoral condyle, potentially causing tears.

Injuries of the muscles and tendons surrounding the knee are caused by acute hyperflexion or hyperextension of the knee or by overuse. These injuries are called strains. Strains are graded similarly to sprains, with first-degree strains stretching muscle or tendon fibers but not tearing them, second-degree strains partially tearing the muscle tendon unit, and third-degree strains completely tearing it.

There can be inflammation of the bursas (known as bursitis: itis=inflammation) of the knee that can occur because of direct blows or chronic use and abuse.

Anatomically, many of the structures that support the knee are interconnected. A knee that is injured may cause damage to one or more structures depending upon the mechanism.

Muscle Tendon Injuries, MCL and LCL Injuries, ACL Injuries and Meniscus Tears

Muscle Tendon Injuries

Almost all of these strains are treated with ice, elevation, and rest. Sometimes compression with an Ace wrap or knee sleeve is recommended, and crutches may be used for a short time to assist with walking. Ibuprofen (Advil, Motrin) or naproxen can be used as an anti-inflammatory medication. (As with all over-the-counter medications, it is important to check with your health care provider or pharmacist regarding safety and drug interactions.)

The mechanism of injury is either hyperextension, in which the hamstring muscles can be stretched or torn, or hyperflexion, in which the quadriceps muscle is injured. Uncommonly, with a hyperflexion injury, the patellar or quadriceps tendon can be damaged and rupture. This injury is characterized by the inability to extend or straighten the knee and a defect that can be felt either above or below the patella (kneecap). Surgery is usually required to repair this injury.

Except for elite athletes, tears of the hamstring muscle are treated conservatively without an operation, allowing time, exercise, and perhaps physical therapy to return the muscle to normal function.

MCL and LCL Injuries

These ligaments can be stretched or torn when the foot is planted and a sideways force is directed to the knee. This can cause significant pain and difficulty walking as the body tries to protect the knee, but there is usually little swelling within the knee. The treatment for this injury may include a hinged knee brace that helps stabilize the knee and control range of motion. RICE (rest, ice, compression, and elevation) are the mainstays of treatment. Surgery may be an option for completely torn ligaments or when the knee joint remains unstable after completing a course of rest and physical therapy. Injuries to these ligaments may also be associated with damage to a meniscus or cruciate ligament.

ACL Injuries

If the foot is planted and there is force applied from the front or back to the knee, then the cruciate ligaments can be damaged. Swelling in the knee occurs within minutes, and attempts at walking are difficult. The definitive diagnosis may be difficult in the emergency department or doctor's office because the swelling and pain make it hard to test knee stability and determine whether the ligament is loose. Health care providers most often confirm the diagnosis by MRI. Long-term treatment may require surgery and significant physical therapy to return good function of the knee joint. Recovery from these injuries is measured in months, not weeks.

Meniscus Tears

The cartilage of the knee can be acutely injured or can gradually tear due to chronic inflammation or arthritis. Acutely, the injury is a twist; the cartilage that is attached to and lays flat on the tibia is pinched between the femoral condyle and the tibial plateau. Pain and swelling occur gradually over many hours (as opposed to an ACL tear which swells much more quickly). Sometimes the injury seems trivial and no care is sought, but chronic pain develops over time. There may be intermittent swelling, pain with walking uphill or climbing steps, or giving way of the knee that results in near falls. Squatting may be painful. History and physical examination often can make the diagnosis, and MRI may be used to confirm it. MRI is also able to define where within the meniscus that the tear has occurred and how much of the cartilage is involved in the tear. This may help guide the decision as to whether surgery, physical therapy, or both would be appropriate.

Fractures, Bursa Inflammation and Patellar Injuries

Fractures

Fractures of the bones of knee are relatively common. The patella, or kneecap, may fracture due to a fall directly onto it or in car accidents, when the knee is driven into the dashboard. If the bone is displaced (pulled apart), surgery may be required for repair, but if the bone is in good position, a knee immobilizer and watchful waiting may be all that is required.

The head of the fibula on the lateral side of the knee joint can be fractured either by a direct blow or as part of an injury to the shin or ankle. This bone usually heals with little intervention, but fractures of this bone can have a major complication. The peroneal nerve wraps around the bone and can be damaged by the fracture. This will cause a foot drop, so do not be surprised if the physician examines your foot when you complain of knee problems.

With jumping injuries, the surface of the tibia can be damaged, resulting in a fracture to the tibial plateau. The mechanism of injury is jumping and landing on a fully extended, straightened knee. Since the femoral condyle sits on the tibial plateau to make the knee joint, it is important that it heals with the most even joint surface as possible to prevent future arthritis and chronic pain. For that reason, after plain X-rays reveal this fracture, a CT scan may be done to make certain that there is no displacement of the bones. This type of fracture may require surgery for repair.

Fractures of the femur require significant force, but in people with osteoporosis, less force is needed to cause a fracture of this large bone. In people with knee replacements who fall, there is a potential weakness at the site of the knee replacement above the femoral condyle, and this can be a site of fracture. The decision to operate or treat by immobilization with a cast will be made by the orthopedist.

Bursa Inflammation

Housemaid's knee (prepatellar bursitis) is due to repetitive kneeling and crawling on the knees. The bursa or space between the skin and kneecap becomes inflamed and fills with fluid. It is a localized injury and does not involve the knee itself. Treatment includes padding the knee and using ibuprofen or naproxen as an anti-inflammatory medication. This injury is commonly seen in carpet installers and roofers. On occasion, if the skin is damaged or torn, this bursa may become infected.

Patellar Injuries

The kneecap sits within the tendon of the quadriceps muscle, in front of the femur, just above the knee joint. It is held in place by the muscles of the knee.

The patella can dislocate laterally (toward the outside of the knee). This occurs more commonly in women because of anatomic differences in the angle aligning the femur and tibia. Fortunately, the dislocation is often returned to the normal position by straightening out the knee, usually resulting in the kneecap popping back into place. Physical therapy for muscle strengthening may be needed to prevent recurrent dislocations. Patellar dislocations are not knee dislocations, which require tearing of three to four major ligaments of the knee. Knee dislocations are uncommon and are a surgical emergency.

Patellofemoral syndrome occurs when the underside of the patella becomes inflamed if irritation develops as the underside of the kneecap rubs against the femoral condyle with each flexion and extension of the knee. This inflammation can cause localized pain, especially with walking down stairs and with running. Treatment includes ice, anti-inflammatory medication, and exercises to balance the quadriceps muscle. More severe cases may require arthroscopic surgery to remove some of the inflamed cartilage and realign parts of the quadriceps muscle.

Risk Factors for Knee Injuries

Accidents happen, and injuries occur on the football field, on the basketball court, on the soccer pitch, and in daily life. Often knee injuries cannot be prevented. Maintaining a healthy weight, keeping fit, staying strong, and stretching may be helpful in minimizing the risk of many injuries, including those that involve the knee.

Imbalances of muscles that surround and support the knee can lead to knee injuries. If either the quadriceps or hamstring muscle groups become weak, the stability of the knee and ability to withstand an injury is decreased.

Similarly, an imbalance between muscles within the quadriceps muscles of the thigh may cause the kneecap (patella) to track improperly, causing patellofemoral syndrome or increasing the risk of patellar dislocation.

Pregnant women are at higher risk for knee injury and pain because of increased weight, the body's shifted center of gravity, and hormonal changes that can weaken ligaments and make them more lax. The knee joint absorbs a significant amount of the force that is generated with each step with walking or running. People who are significantly overweight may develop knee pain because of the excess weight that needs to be supported.

Symptoms and Signs of Knee Injury

Acute knee injuries can cause pain and swelling with difficulty bending the knee and weight-bearing. Acute knee injuries often may be considered as falling into two groups: those where there is almost immediate swelling in the joint associated with the inability to bend the knee and bear weight, and those in which there is discomfort and perhaps localized pain to one side of the knee, but with minimal swelling and minimal effects on walking.

If the swelling occurs immediately, it may suggest a ligament tear or fracture. If the swelling arises over a period of many hours, meniscal or cartilage injuries may be the cause. However, injuries to the knee may involve more than one structure and the symptoms may not present classically.

Longer-term symptoms that point to knee problems will include pain and swelling in addition to other complaints. Inflammation in the joint may be caused by even minor activity. Swelling may be intermittent, brought on by activity, and may gradually resolve as the inflammation decreases.

Pain, too, may come and go. It may not occur right away with activity but might be delayed as the inflammation develops. Pain can also be felt with specific activities. Pain while climbing stairs is a symptom of meniscus injury, where the cartilage is being pinched in the joint as the joint space narrows with knee bending. Pain with walking down stairs suggests patellar pain, where the kneecap is being forced onto the femur.

Giving way, or a feeling of instability of the knee, or popping or grinding in the knee is associated with cartilage or meniscus tears. Locking is the term used when the knee joint refuses to completely straighten, and this is almost always due to torn cartilage. In this situation, the torn piece of cartilage folds upon itself and doesn't allow the knee to extend.

When should you Call the Doctor for a Knee Injury?

Emergent medical care should be sought if, due to injury,

- There is almost immediate swelling in the knee,
- If the bones appear deformed,
- If there is inability to bear weight,

- If the pain is intolerable,
- If there is loss of sensation below the injury site,
- If the foot and ankle turn cold and no pulses can be felt.

Medical care should be considered if a knee injury does not resolve with routine home care, including rest, ice, compression, and elevation (RICE). Other symptoms that may suggest the need for medical care include recurrent pain and swelling.

A swollen joint is never normal, and if it is red and warm or if there is an associated fever, more urgent medical attention should be accessed because of the worry of infection being present. This is particularly a warning sign in infants and children, people who have had knee joint replacements, intravenous drug abusers, and those who have compromised immune systems.

Often, knee injuries are cared for by primary care providers who have the knowledge and skills to diagnose and treat many of the common knee injuries that occur. Orthopedic surgeons are involved in knee injury care to determine whether surgery might be required. They are also the specialists to perform the surgery. Physical therapists have an important role in the treatment of knee injuries regardless of whether surgery is required.

Diagnose of Knee Injuries

The initial evaluation by the health care professional will begin with a medical history. Whether the evaluation is occurring immediately after the injury or weeks later, the physician may ask about the mechanism of injury to help isolate what structures in the knee might be damaged. Is the injury due to a direct blow that might suggest a fracture or contusion (bruise)? Was it a twisting injury that causes a cartilage or meniscus tear? Was there an injury associated with a planted foot to place stress and potentially tear a ligament?

Further questions will address other symptoms. Was swelling present, and if so, did it occur right away or was it delayed by hours? Did the injury prevent weight-bearing or walking? Does going up or down steps cause pain? Is there associated hip or ankle pain? Is this an isolated injury, and have there been other occurrences?

Past medical history and information on medications and allergies will be helpful information to learn about the patient.

Physical examination of the knee begins with inspection, in which the physician will look at the bones and make certain they are where they belong. With fractures of the kneecap or patellar tendon injuries, the kneecap can slide high out of position. Also, patellar dislocations, where the kneecap slides to the outside or lateral part of the knee, are easily evident on inspection. Looking at how the knee is held is also important. If the knee is held slightly flexed, it can be a clue that there is fluid in the joint space, since joint space is maximal at 15 degrees of flexion.

Palpation (feeling) is the next part of the exam, and knowing the anatomy, the physician can feel where any pain might exist and correlate that to the underlying structures like ligaments or muscle-insertion points. Palpation over the joint line, the space between the bones in the front part of the knee, can uncover fluid or tenderness associated with a meniscus injury. This is also the part of the exam when the ligaments are stressed to make certain that they are intact. Sometimes, the physician will also exert stress on the uninjured knee to see how loose or tight the normal ligaments are as a comparison. Finally, the blood supply and nerve supply to the leg and foot will be assessed.

Sometimes X-rays of the knee are required to make certain there are no broken bones, but often with stress or overuse injuries where no direct blow has occurred, plain X-rays may not be initially needed and imaging of the knee may wait until a later date. Standing X-rays of the knees are used to assess the joint space and compare the injured knee to the uninjured one. An MRI might be considered to evaluate the ligaments and cartilage within the knee joint.

Treatments of Knee Injury

Almost all knee injuries will need more than one visit to the doctor. If no operation is indicated, then RICE (rest, ice, compression, and elevation) with some strengthening exercises and perhaps physical therapy will be needed. Sometimes the decision for surgery is delayed to see if the RICE and physical therapy will be effective. Each injury is unique, and treatment decisions depend on what the expectation for function will be. As an example, a torn ACL (anterior cruciate ligament) would usually require surgery in a young athlete or a construction worker, but the ACL may be treated nonoperatively with physical therapy in an 80-year-old who is not very active.

With the technology available, many knee injuries that require surgery can be treated surgically with an arthroscope, in which a camera is used to visualize the damage and small punctures are made in the knee to insert instruments to make repairs. Patients usually begin their post-op rehabilitation within days of the surgery.

If there is no rush to operate, then opportunity exists to pre-hab or strengthen the quadriceps and hamstring muscles beforehand. When a joint like the knee is injured, the muscles around it start to weaken almost immediately. This is also true after the surgery, which can also be considered a further injury. Strong muscles in the preoperative state allow the potential for easier postoperative therapy.

Recovery Time for a Knee Injury

Recovery from a knee injury depends upon the specific injury and can be measured in days to weeks for a sprain to many months to recover from anterior cruciate ligament repair surgery.

Prognosis for a Knee Injury

The goal for treating knee injuries is to return the patient to their previous level of activity. The prognosis for an individual injury depends upon the type of injury, the underlying health of the patient, and their willingness to work with their care provider and therapist to maximize their outcome.

Is it Possible to Prevent Knee Injuries?

Accidents happen, and while many knee injuries occur during recreational activities or sports, more happen at work and at home.

Strong muscles stabilize joints. With the knee, having strong and flexible quadriceps and hamstring muscles can prevent minor stresses to the knee from causing significant injury. Routine stretching exercises or yoga are able to increase muscle flexibility and maintain joint mobility and range of motion.

Proper footwear can also minimize the risk for knee injury. Wearing shoes that are appropriate for the activity can lessen the risk of twisting and other forces that can stress the knee.

ACHILLES TENDON RUPTURE

A total rupture of the Achilles tendon is a complete tear of the tendon and typically affects men over the age of 40. It is not always obvious if you have a completely torn achilles tendon, but if you have, it is essential you seek medical attention as soon as possible.

Achilles Tendon Rupture Symptoms

Symptoms or a torn achilles tendon include:

- A sudden sharp pain in the Achilles tendon at the back of your ankle.
- The pain is often described like being struck physically on the back of your ankle by an object or implement.
- You may hear a loud snapping noise or bang at the time of injury.
- You may see or feel a gap of 4 to 5 cm in your tendon immediately after injury. However, this may be less obvious later as swelling increases.
- You will have considerable loss of function and strength in the injured ankle.
- You will most likely be limping, however, often patients are quite capable of walking or even playing on. This is because other muscles compensate.

Assessment Tests

There are four key tests to help diagnose a complete rupture of the Achilles tendon:

- With the patient lying face down with their feet hanging over the edge of a table or therapy couch, the foot of the injured side will hang directly down, compared to the non injured one would be slightly pointed (plantar flexed).
- Is there a gap of approximately 3 to 6 cm in the Achilles tendon directly after injury? If there is too much swelling then this is not always obvious.
- Plantar flexion strength is significantly reduced. For example, the patient will be unable to point their foot downwards against resistance or go up on top toes.
- Thompson's squeeze test will give a positive result. Thompson's test is performed by squeezing the calf muscles at the belly of the muscle. If the foot does not move then complete rupture is indicated.

Complete Rupture of the Achilles Tendon

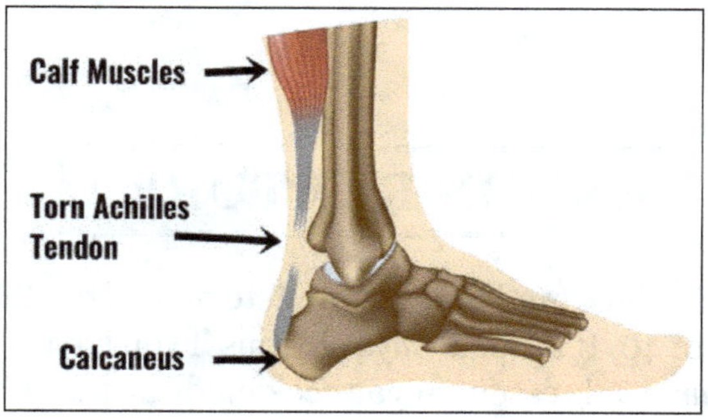

A torn Achilles is simply a tear of the achilles tendon. It can be a partial rupture or a total rupture. A total rupture is 10 times more common in men than in women.

The Achilles tendon connects the calf muscles at the back of the lower leg and inserts at the back of the heel or calcaneus bone. Huge forces are transmitted through the tendon when running and jumping. The tendon itself is surrounded by a thin sheath.

Causes of a Torn Achilles

- Typically it occurs 30 to 40 minutes into a period of exercise, rather than at the start of a session.
- Nearly always it results either from a sudden explosive movement, or when forceably bending the the foot upwards (known as dorsiflexing).
- A rupture may (but not always) follow long term tendon pain which a patient may have put up with, or ignored for some time.

Many patients are able to continue to function following an Achilles rupture due to other lower leg muscles compensating, although the injured leg will be significantly weaker.

ATHLETIC HEART SYNDROME

Athletic heart syndrome is a heart condition that may occur in people who exercise or train for more than an hour a day, most days of the week. Athletic heart syndrome isn't necessarily bad for you if you're an athlete. And it's not what makes young athletes expire in mid-court. While it does lead to structural changes in the heart, a person with the condition usually doesn't notice any symptoms. Athletic heart syndrome doesn't require treatment and is important to diagnose only to rule out heart problems that are serious.

Like any other muscle, the heart gets stronger with exercise. Endurance exercises such as jogging, swimming, and cycling can make the organ bigger, allowing it to pump more blood with every beat. Short, intense workouts such as weight lifting further increase the pumping power by thickening the walls of the heart.

Just as body builders sculpt their abs and biceps into highly unusual shapes, many hard-core, competitive athletes develop extraordinary hearts. Not only is the heart extra large and thick, it also may produce some irregular rhythms (arrhythmia). A person with athletic heart syndrome may also have a markedly slow resting heart rate, in the range of 35 to 50 beats a minute. In addition, electrical impulses can take strange routes across the heart, causing abnormal readings on an electrocardiogram (ECG or EKG). Together, these changes produced by exercise are called athletic heart syndrome.

Is Athletic Heart Syndrome Dangerous?

An enlarged heart, arrhythmia, and unusual ECG readings would all be signs of serious trouble for the average person. In fact, the rhythms and ECG readings associated with athletic heart syndrome often mimic life-threatening disorders. But athletic heart syndrome itself is harmless. The "abnormal" changes in the athlete's heart are actually a testament to the body's ability to adapt.

If an athlete has symptoms of chest pain, reports irregular beats, or has passed out, he or she should get a medical exam to pinpoint the problem. Your doctor may want to run extra tests to determine whether the symptoms are a normal sign of your body's ability to adapt to training, or whether there's some abnormality in your heart. These tests may include an electrocardiogram, sonogram (a picture of the heart using sound waves), or another type of test.

Of course, some athletes really do have heart trouble. Occasionally, seemingly healthy young basketball or football players drop dead in the middle of a game or a practice. In almost every case, doctors trace the death to an unsuspected condition, such as congenital heart disease, but one that has nothing to do with athletic heart syndrome.

How is Athletic Heart Syndrome Treated?

Since athletic heart syndrome is harmless, there's no reason to treat it unless you experience regular light-headedness, chest pains, or you lose consciousness. If you really want a "normal" heart again, all you have to do is stop exercising. Soon, your heart, along with the rest of your body, will sag back into its former shape. But why not keep everything extra strong and healthy for a while? You should be proud of your athletic body, heart included.

PATELLAR TENDINITIS

When it comes to sports like basketball and volleyball, athletes spend a lot of time jumping as they attempt to get balls in - or over - nets. Knees take a lot of stress, particularly for athletes playing in competitive sports. In fact, activities that require running and jumping exert a force on the knees of up to nine to 11 times one's body weight. All that jumping can cause a knee injury known as patellar tendonitis or jumper's knee.

Patellar tendonitis is a chronic overuse injury to the patellar tendon. The injury, commonly found in people who play basketball or volleyball, causes inflammation as a result of chronic, repetitive jumping and excessive exertion of the knees.

Left untreated, jumper's knee can result in prolonged pain during and after the activity and an inability to perform at a high level. The repetitive stress of continued play can lead to micro-tears or a complete rupture of the patellar tendon. If this happens, surgery is required to repair the tendon.

Surgery for patellar tendonitis is a last resort. It is best to recognize and treat the condition early to minimize lost time due to the injury.

Patellar Tendonitis Symptoms

- Patella (kneecap) laxity or an unstable patella, which includes pain, swelling and inflammation of the kneecap.
- Hamstring tightness, indicated by poor flexibility in the back of the thigh.
- Hamstring tightness, indicated by poor flexibility in the back of the thigh.
- Heel cord/achilles tendon tightness, which is identified by poor flexibility in the rear of the ankle.

- Muscular asymmetry, or disparity between muscle size in legs, which can cause muscle shrinkage.
- Ankle dorsi flexion weakness, which affects the muscles around the ankle.

To prevent patellar tendonitis, athletes should have a thorough pre- mid- and post-season strength and conditioning exercise program, as well as maintain lower extremity flexibility.

Weight lifting and cardiovascular workouts are good methods of avoiding jumper's knee.

Patellar Tendonitis Treatment

Treatment for jumper's knee involves resting, applying ice to the injury, compressing the injury and elevating the affected area. According to Cooper, the letters R-E-S-T explain how best to rest after a jumper's knee injury.

'R' stands for rehabilitation, 'E' stands for exercises prescribed by a physician, 'S' stands for strength and endurance training and 'T' stands for time off from the activity that caused the injury. The athlete can still use many machines in the gym or ride a bicycle. You want to stay active to avoid muscle atrophy.

In addition, an over-the-counter anti-inflammatory, such as ibuprofen, is used as part of the treatment. Athletes can run a risk of re-injury if they do not participate in strength and conditioning exercises.

Individualized Treatment Approach

Each individual with patellar tendonitis must be approached differently. Treatment depends on the phase of the injury, whether it is acute or chronic. There is no timeline in recovering from jumper's knee - recovery may take a week for one person and a month for someone else.

Jumper's knee is most often found in adults aged 30 or older, especially those "weekend athletes" who do not regularly do strength and conditioning exercises.

The condition is also frequently found in children ages 10-16 because their muscles are still growing and developing.

FEMALE ATHLETE TRIAD

Sports and exercise are part of a balanced, healthy lifestyle. People who play sports are healthier; get better grades; are less likely to experience depression; and use alcohol, cigarettes, and drugs less frequently than people who aren't athletes. But for some girls, not balancing the needs of their bodies and their sports can have major consequences.

Some girls who play sports or exercise intensely are at risk for a problem called female athlete triad. Female athlete triad is a combination of three conditions: disordered eating, amenorrhea, and osteoporosis. A female athlete can have one, two, or all three parts of the triad.

Disordered Eating

Most girls with female athlete triad try to lose weight as a way to improve their athletic performance. The disordered eating that accompanies female athlete triad can range from not eating enough calories to keep up with energy demands to avoiding certain types of food the athlete thinks are "bad" (such as foods containing fat) to serious eating disorders like anorexia nervosa or bulimia nervosa.

Amenorrhea

Exercising intensely and not eating enough calories can lead to decreases in the hormones that help regulate the menstrual cycle. As a result, a girl's periods may become irregular or stop altogether. Of course, it's normal for teens to occasionally miss periods, especially in the first year. A missed period does not automatically mean female athlete triad. It could mean something else is going on, like pregnancy or a medical condition. If you are having sex and miss your period, talk to your doctor.

Some girls who participate intensively in sports may never even get their first period because they've been training so hard. Others may have had periods, but once they increase their training and change their eating habits, their periods may stop.

Osteoporosis

Estrogen is lower in girls with female athlete triad. Low estrogen levels and poor nutrition, especially low calcium intake, can lead to osteoporosis, the third aspect of the triad. Osteoporosis is a weakening of the bones due to the loss of bone density and improper bone formation. This condition can ruin a female athlete's career because it may lead to stress fractures and other injuries.

Usually, the teen years are a time when girls should be building up their bone mass to their highest levels — called peak bone mass. Not getting enough calcium now can also have a lasting effect on how strong a woman's bones are later in life.

Who Gets Female Athlete Triad?

Many girls have concerns about the size and shape of their bodies. But being a highly competitive athlete and participating in a sport that requires you to train extra hard can increase that worry.

Girls with female athlete triad often care so much about their sports that they would do almost anything to improve their performance. Martial arts and rowing are examples of sports that classify athletes by weight class, so focusing on weight becomes an important part of the training program and can put a girl at risk for disordered eating.

Participation in sports where a thin appearance is valued can also put a girl at risk for female athlete triad. Sports such as gymnastics, figure skating, diving, and ballet are examples of sports that value a thin, lean body shape. Some athletes may even be told by coaches or judges that losing weight would improve their scores.

Even in sports where body size and shape aren't as important, such as distance running and cross-country skiing, girls may be pressured by teammates, parents, partners, and coaches who mistakenly believe that "losing just a few pounds" could improve their performance.

The truth is, losing those few pounds generally doesn't improve performance at all. People who are fit and active enough to compete in sports generally have more muscle than fat, so it's the muscle that gets starved when a girl cuts back on food. Plus, if a girl loses weight when she doesn't need to, it interferes with healthy body processes such as menstruation and bone development.

In addition, for some competitive female athletes, problems such as low self-esteem, a tendency toward perfectionism, and family stress place them at risk for disordered eating.

Signs and Symptoms

If a girl has risk factors for female athlete triad, she may already be experiencing some symptoms and signs of the disorder, such as:

- Weight loss.
- No periods or irregular periods.
- Fatigue and decreased ability to concentrate.
- Stress fractures (fractures that occur even if a person hasn't had a significant injury).
- Other injuries.

Girls with female athlete triad often have signs and symptoms of eating disorders, such as:

- Continued dieting in spite of weight loss.
- Preoccupation with food and weight.
- Frequent trips to the bathroom during and after meals.
- Using laxatives.
- Brittle hair or nails.
- Dental cavities because in girls with bulimia tooth enamel is worn away by frequent vomiting.

- Sensitivity to cold.
- Low heart rate and blood pressure.
- Heart irregularities and chest pain.

How Doctors Help?

An extensive physical examination is a crucial part of diagnosing female athlete triad. A doctor who thinks a girl has female athlete triad will probably ask questions about her periods, her nutrition and exercise habits, any medications she takes, and her feelings about her body. This is called the medical history.

Poor nutrition can also affect the body in many ways, so a doctor might order blood tests to check for anemia and other problems associated with the triad. The doctor also will check for medical reasons why a girl may be losing weight and missing her periods. Because osteoporosis can put someone at higher risk for bone fractures, the doctor may also request tests to measure bone density.

Doctors don't work alone to help a girl with female athlete triad. Coaches and trainers, parents, physical therapists, pediatricians and adolescent medicine specialists, sports medicine doctors, nutritionists and dietitians, and mental health specialists can all work together to treat the physical and emotional problems that a girl with female athlete triad faces.

It might be tempting to shrug off several months of missed periods, but getting help right away is important. In the short term, female athlete triad may lead to reduced physical performance, stress fractures, and other injuries. Over the long term, it can cause bone weakness, long-term effects on the reproductive system, and heart problems.

A girl who is recovering from female athlete triad might work with a dietitian to help reach and maintain a healthy weight while eating enough calories and nutrients for health and good athletic performance. Depending on how much the girl is exercising, she may have to reduce the length of her workouts. Talking to a psychologist or therapist can help her deal with depression, pressure from coaches or family members, or low self-esteem and can help her find ways to deal with her problems other than restricting food intake or exercising excessively.

Some girls may need to take hormones to supply their bodies with estrogen to help prevent further bone loss. Calcium and vitamin D supplementation can also help when someone has bone loss as the result of female athlete triad.

Tips for Female Athletes

Here are a few tips to help teen athletes stay on top of their physical condition:

- Keep track of your periods. It's easy to forget when you had your last visit from Aunt Flo, so keep track of your periods on a calendar and mark down when your period starts and stops and if the bleeding is particularly heavy or light. That way, if you start missing periods, you'll know right away and you'll have accurate information to give to your doctor.

- Don't skip meals or snacks. If you're constantly on the go between school, practice, and competitions you may be tempted to skip meals and snacks to save time. But eating now will improve performance later, so stock your locker or bag with quick and easy favorites such as bagels, string cheese, unsalted nuts and seeds, raw vegetables, granola bars, and fruit.
- Visit a dietitian or nutritionist who works with teen athletes. He or she can help you get your dietary game plan into gear and find out if you're getting enough calories and key nutrients such as iron, calcium, and protein. And if you need supplements, a nutritionist can recommend the best choices.
- Do it for you. Pressure from teammates, parents, or coaches can turn a fun activity into a nightmare. If you're not enjoying your sport, make a change. Remember: It's your body and your life. You — not your coach or teammates — will have to live with any damage you do to your body now.

RELATIVE ENERGY DEFICIENCY IN SPORT

Relative energy deficiency in sport (RED-S) is a syndrome in which disordered eating (or low energy availability), amenorrhoea/oligomenorrhoea, and decreased bone mineral density (osteoporosis and osteopenia) are present. RED-S is the broader, more comprehensive name for what was formerly known as female athlete triad (or simply the triad), which was a condition seen in females participating in sports that emphasize leanness or low body weight. As it was also seen in males, the name was changed to the comprehensive term RED-S. The triad is a serious illness with lifelong health consequences and can potentially be fatal.

Classification

The female athlete triad is a syndrome of three interrelated conditions. Thus, if an athlete is suffering from one element of the triad, it is likely that she is suffering from the other two components of the triad as well. With the increase in female participation in sports, the incidence of a triad of disorders particular to women—the female athlete triad—has also increased. The female athlete triad and its relationship with athletics was identified in the 1980s as the prevalence increased during this period, and symptoms, risk factors, causes, and treatments were studied in depth and their relatedness evaluated. The condition is most common in cross country running, gymnastics, and figure skating. Many of those who suffer from the triad are involved in some sort of athletics, in order to promote weight loss and leanness. The competitive sports that promote this physical leanness may result in disordered eating and be responsible for the origin of the female athlete triad. For some women, the disorder can have major health consequences. In addition, for some competitive female athletes, problems such as low self-esteem, a tendency toward perfectionism, and family stress place them at risk for disordered eating.

Signs and Symptoms

Clinical symptoms of the Triad may include disordered eating, fatigue, hair loss, cold hands and feet, dry skin, noticeable weight loss, increased healing time from injuries (e.g., lingering bruises), increased incidence of bone fracture and cessation of menses. Affected females may also struggle with low self-esteem and depression.

Upon physical examination, a physician may also note the following symptoms: elevated carotene in the blood, anemia, orthostatic hypotension, electrolyte irregularities, hypoestrogenism, vaginal atrophy, and bradycardia.

An athlete may show signs of restrictive eating, but not meet the clinical criteria for an eating disorder. She may also display subtle menstrual disturbances, such as a change in menstrual cycle length, anovulation, or luteal phase defects, but not yet have developed complete amenorrhea. Likewise, an athlete's bone density may decrease, but may not yet have dropped below her age-matched normal range. These signs can be considered "occult," as no one symptom may be severe enough to seek medical attention, leaving the Triad to go unnoticed or untreated.

Disordered Eating

Energy availability is defined as energy intake minus energy expended. Energy is taken in through food consumption. Our bodies expend energy through normal functioning as well as through exercise. In the case of female athlete triad, low energy availability may be due to eating disorders, but not necessarily so. Athletes may experience low energy availability by exercising more without a concomitant change in eating habits, or they may increase their energy expenditure while also eating less. Disordered eating is defined among this situation due to the low caloric intake or low energy availability.

While most athletes do not meet the clinical criteria to be diagnosed with an eating disorder such as anorexia nervosa or bulimia nervosa, many will exhibit disordered eating habits such as fasting, as well as avoiding certain types of food the athlete thinks are "bad" (such as foods containing fat). More severe examples of disordered eating habits may include binge-eating; purging; and the use of diet-pills, laxatives, diuretics, and enemas.

By restricting their diet, the athlete may worsen their problem of low energy availability. Having low dietary energy from excessive exercise and/or dietary restrictions leaves too little energy for the body to carry out normal functions such as maintaining a regular menstrual cycle or healthy bone density.

Amenorrhea

Amenorrhea, defined as the cessation of a woman's menstrual cycle for more than three months, is the second disorder in the Triad. Weight fluctuations from dietary restrictions and/or excessive exercise affect the hypothalamus's output of gonadotropic hormones. Gonadotropic hormones "stimulate growth of the gonads and the secretion of sex hormones." (e.g. gonadotropin-releasing hormone, lutenizing hormone and follicle stimulating hormone.) These gonadotropic hormones play a role in stimulating estrogen release from the ovaries. Without estrogen release, the menstrual cycle is disrupted. Exercising intensely and not eating enough calories can lead to decreases in estrogen, the hormone that helps to regulate the menstrual cycle. As a result, periods may become irregular or stop altogether.

There are two types of amenorrhea. A woman who has been having her period and then stops menstruating for ninety days or more is said to have secondary amenorrhea. In the case of RED-S, the majority of secondary amenorrhea cases are attributed to Functional Hypothalamic Amenorrhea (FHA), an adaptive mechanism to preserve energy for survival and vital processes rather than reproduction when energy balance is low. Primary amenorrhea is characterized by delayed menarche (the onset of menses during puberty). Delayed menarche may be associated with delay of the development of secondary sexual characteristics.

Osteoporosis

Osteoporosis is defined by the National Institutes of Health as "a skeletal disorder characterized by compromised bone strength predisposing a person to an increased risk of fracture." Low estrogen levels and poor nutrition, especially low calcium intake, can lead to osteoporosis, the third aspect of the triad. This condition can ruin a female athlete's career because it may lead to stress fractures and other injuries.

Patients with female athlete triad get osteoporosis due to hypoestrogenemia, or low estrogen levels. With estrogen deficiency, the osteoclasts live longer and are therefore able to resorb more bone. In response to the increased bone resorption, there is increased bone formation and a high-turnover state develops which leads to bone loss and perforation of the trabecular plates. As osteoclasts break down bone, patients see a loss of bone mineral density. Low bone mineral density renders bones more brittle and hence susceptible to fracture. Because athletes are active and their bones must endure mechanical stress, the likelihood of experiencing bone fracture is particularly high.

Additionally, because those suffering with female athlete triad are also restricting their diet, they may also not be consuming sufficient amounts vitamins and minerals which contribute to bone density; not getting enough calcium or vitamin D further exacerbates the problem of weak bones.

Bone mass is now thought to peak between the ages of 18-25. Thus, behaviors which result in low bone density in youth could be detrimental to an athlete's bone health throughout her lifetime.

In addition, ovulation is the primary way that females create the hormone progesterone. When an ovum is released from the ovary, the structure that remains develops into the corpus luteum. The corpus luteum emits the hormone progesterone during the 10-16 days of the luteal phase. Without experiencing regular, ovulatory menstrual cycles, the female is not secreting the hormone progesterone during the luteal phase of her cycle. Progesterone directly stimulates osteoblasts to make new bone. Therefore if the woman is not ovulating, she is not creating progesterone, and misses out on this opportunity to stimulate new bone growth.

Causes

Gymnastics, figure skating, ballet, diving, swimming, and long distance running are examples of sports which emphasize low body weight. The Triad is seen more often in aesthetic sports such as these versus ball game sports. Women taking part in these sports may be at an increased risk for developing female athlete triad.

Athletes at greatest risk for low energy availability are those who restrict dietary energy intake, who exercise for prolonged periods, who are vegetarian, and who limit the types of food they will eat. Many factors appear to contribute to disordered eating behaviors and clinical eating disorders. Dieting is a common entry point and interest has focused on the contribution of environmental and social factors, psychological predisposition, low self-esteem, family dysfunction, abuse, biological factors, and genetics. Additional factors for athletes include early start of sport-specific training and dieting, injury, and a sudden increase in training volume. Surveys show more negative eating attitude scores in athletic disciplines favoring leanness. Disordered eating behaviors are risk factors for eating disorders.

Treatment

The underlying cause of the female athlete triad is an imbalance between energy taken into the body (through nutrition) and energy used by the body (through exercise). The treatment includes correcting this imbalance by either increasing calories in a diet or by decreasing calories burned by exercise for 12 months or longer. Persons with female athlete triad should get treatment from a multi-disciplinary team that includes a physician, dietitian, and mental health counselor, and seek support from family, friends, and their coach.

Because a symptom of the female athlete triad is menstrual dysfunction, some physicians may recommend oral contraceptives because those pills will regulate the menstrual cycle. However, the underlying cause of the menstrual disorder is an energy imbalance, and using pills to regulate the menstrual cycle without changes in diet and behavior is likely to mask the food deficiency and delay appropriate treatment. A woman taking contraceptives to treat menstrual dysfunction without correcting this energy imbalance will continue to lose bone density.

Less Exercise

Continued participation in training and competition depends on the physical and mental health of the athlete. Athletes who weigh less than 80 percent of their ideal body weight may not be able to safely participate.

Persons with female athlete triad are often asked by health care providers to reduce the amount of time they spend exercising by 10-12 percent.

Eating More

Low energy availability with or without eating disorders, functional hypothalamic amenorrhea, and osteoporosis, alone or in combination, pose significant health risks to physically active girls and women. Prevention, recognition, and treatment of these clinical conditions should be a priority of those who work with female athletes to ensure that they maximize the benefits of regular exercise.

Patients are recommended to work with a dietician who can monitor their nutritional status and help the patient work towards a healthy goal weight. Patients should also meet with a psychiatrist or psychologist to address the psychological aspects of the triad. Therefore, it is important that trainers and coaches are made aware of the athlete's condition and be part of her recovery.

Medicine

Patients are also sometimes treated pharmacologically. To both induce menses and improve bone density, doctors may prescribe cyclic estrogen or progesterone as is used to treat post-menopausal women. Patients may also be put on oral contraceptives to stimulate regular periods. In addition to hormone therapy, nutrition supplements may be recommended. Doctors may prescribe calcium supplements. Vitamin D supplements may be also used because this vitamin aids in calcium absorption. Bisphosphonates and calcitonin, used to treat adults with osteoporosis, may be prescribed, although their effectiveness in adolescents has not yet been established. Finally, if indicated by a psychiatric examination, the affected athlete may be prescribed anti-depressants and in some cases benzodiazepines to help in alleviating severe distress at mealtimes.

Prognosis

Sustained low energy availability, with or without disordered eating, can impair health. Psychological problems associated with eating disorders include low self-esteem, depression, and anxiety disorders. Medical complications involve the cardiovascular, endocrine, reproductive, skeletal, gastrointestinal, renal, and central nervous systems. The prognosis for anorexia nervosa is grave with a six-fold increase in standard mortality rates compared to the general population. In one study, 5.4% of athletes with eating disorders reported suicide attempts. Although 83% of anorexia nervosa patients partially recover, the rate of sustained recovery of weight, menstrual function and eating behavior is only 33%.

Amenorrheic women can be infertile, due to the absence of ovarian follicular development, ovulation, and luteal function. Consequences of hypoestrogenism seen in amenorrheic athletes include impaired endothelium-dependent arterial vasodilation, which reduces the perfusion of working muscle, impaired skeletal muscle oxidative metabolism, elevated low-density lipoprotein cholesterol levels, and vaginal dryness.

Due to low bone mineral density that declines as the number of missed menstrual cycles accumulates, and the loss of BMD may not be fully reversible. Stress fractures occur more commonly in physically active women with menstrual irregularities and/or low BMD with a relative risk for stress fracture two to four times greater in amenorrheic than eumenorrheic athletes. Fractures also occur in the setting of nutritional deficits and low BMD.

References

- Ankle-injury, injury-fact-sheets, resources-advice: sma.org.au, Retrieved 20 June, 2019
- Joy, Elizabeth (2009-03-15). "Health-Related Concerns of the Female Athlete". American Family Physician. 79 (6): 489–495. Retrieved 14 March 2012
- Sprained-ankle, acute-ankle-injuries, ankle-pain, sport-injuries: sportsinjuryclinic.net, Retrieved 21 July, 2019
- Seifert-Klauss, V.; Prior, J. C. (2010). "Progesterone and Bone: Actions Promoting Bone Health in Women". Journal of Osteoporosis. 2010: 1–18. Doi:10.4061/2010/845180. PMC 2968416. PMID 21052538
- Ankle-sprain-taping, acute-ankle-injuries, acute-ankle-injuries, sport-injuries: sportsinjuryclinic.net, Retrieved 22 January, 2019
- Seifert-Klauss, V.; Prior, J. C. (2010). "Progesterone and Bone: Actions Promoting Bone Health in Women". Journal of Osteoporosis. 2010: 1–18. Doi:10.4061/2010/845180. PMC 2968416. PMID 21052538
- Groin-strain, groin-pain, hip-groin, sport-injuries: sportsinjuryclinic.net, Retrieved 23 February, 2019
- Shin-Pain, Pages, sports-injuries, injuries-emergencies, health-issues, English: healthychildren.org, Retrieved 24 March, 2019

Sport-Specific Injuries and their Treatment

CHAPTER 3

There are some injuries that are specific to particular sports such as ankle injuries in basketball, and sprains, fractures and concussions in baseball. This chapter has been carefully written to provide an easy understanding of different sports-specific injuries such as injuries related to football, swimming and racquet sports.

BASKETBALL INJURIES

According to the American Orthopaedic Society for Sports Medicine (AOSSM) Sports Trauma and Overuse Prevention (STOP) program, the most common basketball injuries (considering recreational as well as professional venues) are ankle sprains, jammed fingers, knee injuries, deep thigh bruising, facial cuts, and foot fractures. According to a study based upon a 17-year overview of injuries in the NBA:

> "Professional athletes in the NBA experience a high rate of game-related injuries. Patellofemoral inflammation is the most significant problem in terms of days lost in competition, whereas ankle sprains are the most common injury."

While lower limb injuries e.g. ankle sprains, patellofemoral pain syndrome and other knee injuries, and leg/foot stress fractures are the most common ones among NBA players, injuries to the hips, head/face, and wrist/hand join the list of common fairly basketball injuries.

Whether you're playing a pick-up game at the neighborhood recreation center, or contesting for an Olympic gold medal, or on contract with a professional team, or just shooting lay-ups and free-throws in your own driveway you're equally susceptible to the occasional jammed finger or rolled ankle.

Muscle Groups Involved in Playing Basketball

Not surprisingly, it's the muscles and joints most frequently used while playing basketball that are the ones that are most susceptible to injury. So which muscles are these, exactly? Basically, they're the muscles involved in running quickly, jumping high, stopping and starting and cutting on a dime, and passing, catching and shooting the ball.

When sliding side to side, or crouching to defend a player, or lowering the hips into a squat at the beginning of the shooting motion the quadriceps (thighs) and gluteal muscles (hips/buttocks) are primarily involved. Any kind of jumping to launch a jump-shot, or contest for a rebound, or leap to block a shot or intercept a pass requires also the engagement of the calf muscles. The explosiveness of a quick first step utilizes the calves, hamstrings, and quadriceps in tandem.

Shooting, defending, and passing the basketball also involve the muscles of the arms and shoulders: the triceps, biceps, deltoids, and rotator cuff. The triceps in particular factor into the ability to shoot effectively from a distance (say from 3-point range). And the chest and back muscles the pectoralis and trapezius also are centrally involved in these movements.

Also of vital importance are the muscles of the core: It's the strength of the abdominal, oblique, psoas, pelvic floor, and lower-back muscles that provide an efficient foundation for changing directions quickly, and making sharp cuts. A strong core also allows for a stable defensive stance, and an overall sense of balance and ease of movement.

Given that pretty much every muscle group of the body is involved in playing basketball, a strength training program that addresses each of these muscle groups will, in a general way, help to prevent injury.

Common Basketball Injuries: Treatment and Prevention

Now let's explore some specific injuries that are common for basketball players, including tips on how best to prevent them along with basic treatment strategies. We'll begin with the most common of all basketball injuries: the ankle sprain.

Basketball Injuries to the Foot and Ankle

An ankle sprain happens when you twist, roll, or turn your ankle in an awkward way, which results in the stretching or tearing of one or more of the ligaments in the ankle. Such an injury typically results in pain, swelling, and stiffness (i.e. limited range of motion) in the ankle and can take days, weeks, or months to fully heal, depending upon the severity.

Among NBA players, it's the Golden State Warrior's Stephen Curry whose frequent ankle sprains resolved at least in part via surgery and an intensive and ongoing training regimen (focused in large part on core strengthening) have been most impactful. When Curry is healthy, his impact on a given game is almost immeasurable. But there was a time when his career was genuinely in jeopardy, because of the seriousness and frequency of this most common of basketball injuries.

Treatment for ankle sprains: The basic RICE protocol: rest, ice, compression, and elevation. If the symptoms don't resolve within a few days, an x-ray and evaluation by a physician may be required. Once the immediate symptoms have diminished, physical therapy exercises can support a full recovery.

Prevention of ankle sprains: Along with core strengthening (Steph Curry's 1 strategy), proper equipment is vital. Wear indoor basketball shoes that prevent slipping, and provide adequate support for the ankles. Ankle braces and/or taping can be used for additional support, particularly if you're prone to ankle sprains.

Other foot/ankle injuries: Stress fractures are another common basketball injury, particularly in the foot and lower leg (tibia). These are treated initially via immobilization and temporary ceasing of weight-bearing activities; with return to play happening only once the fracture has healed completely.

Basketball Injuries to the Hip and Thigh

Deep thigh bruising (contusion) is another common basketball injury, typically caused by an opponent's elbow or knee inadvertently striking a player's thigh muscles. However, among NBA players it has been the quadriceps tendinopathy suffered by Kawhi Leonard which has been the thigh injury with the greatest impact on the league. Conflict regarding the treatment (or mistreatment) of this injury during the 2017-18 season resulted eventually in Leonard being traded from the San Antonio Spurs to the Toronto Raptors.

Treatment of thigh bruising: As with ankle sprains, the initial treatment includes rest, ice, compression, and elevation (RICE). Once the acute symptoms have subsided, light training with physical therapy can bridge a player's journey back to full activity.

Prevention of thigh bruising: Injuries such as this often can't be prevented. However, having a comprehensive yoga or stretching program along with weight training can lesson the impact of the injury. Also, compression sleeves and/or girdles with thigh pads can be worn for additional protection.

Basketball Injuries to the Knee.

As mentioned above, patellofemoral pain syndrome pain felt behind the kneecap, where the kneecap (patella) meets the thigh bone (femur) is one of the most common knee injuries among basketball players. The pain is generally the result of excessive joint pressure due to poor kneecap alignment, which affects the joint surface behind the kneecap.

Treatment for patellofemoral pain syndrome: Once again, the initial treatment is rest (avoiding activities that cause pain), ice, compression, and elevation. Once pain and inflammation is reduced, correcting the biomechanical imbalances that created the problem is the next step toward full recovery.

Prevention of patellofemoral pain syndrome: Normalize muscle balance and establish proper biomechanics, through physical therapy, yoga, or pilates. Wearing a therapeutic compression sleeve or knee brace can also be beneficial.

Other knee injuries: Unfortunately, more serious knee injuries while not as common as patellofemoral pain syndrome are not entirely uncommon among basketball players, so are worth mentioning. The Boston Celtic's Kyrie Irving suffered a fractured kneecap, and complications from this injury prevented him from joining his team in the 2018 NBA playoffs. And the New York Knicks 7-foot 3-inch all-star forward Kristaps Porzingas suffered a torn ACL (anterior cruciate ligament) in February 2018 which is an injury that can take up to a year or more to fully resolve. Both of these players are leaders of their team, and so their absence was deeply felt.

The best strategy for preventing a serious knee injury is to maintain balanced strength in the muscles of your legs, which support the knees. Commit to doing a yoga, pilates or stretching routine prior to practices and games, to maintain proper biomechanics. (The yoga pose Hero Pose (virasana) is particularly excellent for overall knee health.) A knee brace can provide additional support and protection.

Basketball Injuries to the Wrist and Hand.

It should come as no surprise given all the passing and catching of the basketball, not to mention attempted steals, etc. that jammed fingers are one of the most common injuries. Instead of landing snug in the palm of your hand, the ball hits the tip of a finger, jamming the finger into one of its joints, creating pain and swelling. Happily, the solution is usually pretty simply, and recovery time modest.

Treatment of jammed fingers: Apply ice, and then "buddy tape" the injured finger to the adjacent finger. This helps protect the finger while it heals, and may also allow you to return to the game, if the injury isn't serious. If pain and swelling haven't resolved after a few days, an x-ray and evaluation by a trainer or physician may be required.

Prevention of jammed finger: Preventing jammed fingers is about mindfulness as much as anything else. Follow the ball visually all the way into your hands before doing what you're going to do next, i.e. dibbling, shooting, or passing. When you don't have the ball, keep your vision wide and soft, maintaining awareness of all the players on the floor, as well as the ball. This will make it less likely that you'll be surprised by the ball arriving in your hands.

Other injuries to the wrist and hand: The Phoenix Sun's Devon Booker who once scored 70 points in a game recently had surgery to repair the fifth metacarpophalangeal joint in his right hand. There are also hand injuries that basketball players pick up in ways that are only tangentially related to actual basketball activity: Lebron James, for instance, injured his hand via punching a blackboard, out of frustration after losing a game in the 2018 playoffs. And the Boston Celtic's Marcus Smart (not very smartly) punched a glass frame, cutting his hand seriously and just narrowly missing severing a couple of tendons.

Basketball injuries to the Head and Face.

Cuts are the most common basketball injury to the head and face. In the game where he broke the NBA record for made 3-point shots, shooting guard Klay Thompson accidentally knocked heads with his Golden State Warriors teammate Damian Jones, resulting in a cut on his forehead that required stitches. Luckily, most such cuts are not serious.

Treatment of cuts: Clean and disinfect the cut, and apply "butterfly" sterile tape to temporarily suture it. If the cut is deeper, it may require stitches. Apply ice if there is pain or swelling. As with any head injury, be on the lookout for concussion symptoms. If an NBA player is experiencing these, he'll be placed in the league's concussion protocol.

Prevention: Cuts to the head or face resulting from collisions can't really be prevented, though training to enhance proprioception might increase your chances of avoiding such collisions.

BASEBALL INJURIES

Baseball injuries tend to usually occur in the shoulder and elbow, due to the high forces involved. This is especially true in pitchers, but other positions, as well as batters, may also suffer from this kind of injury.

Medial ligament injuries at the elbow are the most common injuries in pitchers. This is damage to the ligament on the inside of the elbow, caused by repeated stress. Golfer's elbow is another injury which is common and is sometimes actually called throwers elbow. It is a degenerative condition of the tendons of the forearm muscles where they attach to the inner elbow.

Here are the six most common baseball injuries.

Rotator Cuff Injuries

Rotator cuff strain is a tear to any of the four rotator cuff muscles in the shoulder. These muscles are important for stabilizing the shoulder joint. Symptoms of a torn rotator cuff will usually consist of sudden pain in the shoulder sometimes accompanied by a tearing feeling. This can be severe and may transmit down into the arm.

Impingement Syndrome

Impingement syndrome of the shoulder is sometimes called swimmer's shoulder or thrower's shoulder and is caused by the tendons of the rotator cuff becoming impinged as they pass through the shoulder joint. Symptoms include shoulder pain which comes on gradually over a period of time.

Shoulder Instability

Shoulder subluxation or shoulder instability occurs when the shoulder partially dislocates. The shoulder joint by its nature allows a large range of movement which means it is likely to be less stable. It may be associated with pain and or dead arm sensation.

Medial Elbow Ligament Sprain

Medial elbow ligament sprain – The medial collateral (MCL) ligament of the elbow is situated on the inner elbow and helps to provide stability to the joint. Damage to this ligament can occur through an impact injury or an accident or from repetitive overuse, for example throwing with poor technique.

Golfer's Elbow

Throwers elbow (Golfers elbow) or medial epicondylitis is an injury similar to tennis elbow but causing pain on the inside of the elbow instead. It is sometimes known as throwers elbow. Symptoms often come on gradually through overuse although acute injuries can occur to pitchers who throw too hard too soon or with bad technique.

Tennis Elbow

Tennis elbow also known as lateral epicondylitis, is a condition causing pain on the outside of the elbow. Symptoms usually come on gradually through overuse.

Immediate First Aid for Acute Injuries

The PRICE principles are the gold standard set for treating acute sports injuries. The acronym stands for Protection, Rest, Ice, Compression and Elevation and should be applied as early as possible and continued for at least the first 24-72 hours.

Protection

Protection of the damaged tissue is vital to prevent further damage and enable the healing process to start efficiently and effectively. There are a number of ways to protect the injured area all with the same aim of limiting further movement and use of the joint/muscle/ligament/tendon. One way this can be achieved is by using a support or splint.

Rest

In the early stages, rest is one of the most important components of the P.R.I.C.E principle but is often neglected or ignored. It does not only refer to the prolonged period of time that the athlete will be out of action but also to the immediate period after the injury.

An athlete must know when to stop training and allow the injured area to heal otherwise repetitive minor injuries can often result in a more severe injury that keeps the athlete out for much longer.

If an injury is sustained during sporting activity some athletes have a tendency to 'run it off'. This implies that by continuing to participate in the exercise, the injury will simply go away. In fact, in the majority of cases, this is not true and is not advisable.

Ice

Ice therapy, also known as cryotherapy, is one of the most widely known and used treatment modalities for acute sports injuries. It is cheap, easy to use and requires very little time to or expertise to prepare.

The application of ice to an injury, in the acute phase, can substantially decrease the extent of the damage. It achieves this in a number of different ways:

- Decreases the amount of bleeding by closing down the blood vessels (called vasoconstriction).
- Reduces pain (pain gate theory).
- Reduces muscle spasm.
- Reduces the risk of cell death (also called necrosis) by decreasing the rate of metabolism.

Ice is usually applied to the injured site by means of a bag filled with crushed ice which is wrapped in a damp towel. The damp towel is essential as it forms a barrier between the bag of ice and the skin and reduces the risk of an "ice burn". do not leave the ice on for more than 15 minutes as you could cause an "ice burn".

There are a small number of areas that you should not apply ice to which include the neck, the outside bone of the elbow, the collarbone (upper end), the front of the hip (bony part) and the outer bone of the knee. The reason for this is there is a superficial nerve just below the skin in these areas that can be damaged by applying ice to it. Always check for contraindications.

Compression

Applying compression to an injured area minimises the amount of swelling that forms after an injury in two ways and should be applied for the first 24 to 72 hours from the onset of injury. Compression can be applied through a number of methods. The most effective of these is by using a compression bandage which is an elasticated bandage that simply fits around the affected limb.

Elevation

Elevation of the injured limb is the final principle of PRICE but is equally as important as the other 4. Elevation allows gravity to drain the fluid away from the injured site. This aids in decreasing the swelling which in turn may decrease the pain associated with the oedema (swelling).

Professional Treatment

If you have any of the following symptoms you should seek further medical assistance.

- Severe pain, especially on walking.
- Severe swelling (oedema).
- Altered sensation in the foot – such as a feeling of "pins and needles" (paresthesia) or a "loss of feeling" (anaesthesia).
- Unable to complete normal daily activities after the initial 72 hours.

Further medical assistance can be sought through either your local GP or a private clinician such as a podiatrist, physiotherapist, sports therapist, osteopath or chiropractor. If you have followed the P.R.I.C.E. principles and are still unable to walk after 72 hours or still have severe pain that is not subsiding after the first 72 hours you should visit your local A&E department for further assessment.

Secondly, if you have applied for P.R.I.C.E. principles and still have weakness that lasts a long time (more than 2 weeks) or have ongoing discomfort in your foot or heel, you are highly recommended to seek advice from a specialist expert – such as a podiatrist or physiotherapist, osteopath, or chiropractor – who can provide you with advice and an appropriate and effective recovery and rehabilitation program.

Baseball Injury Prevention

Injury prevention strategies are very similar in most sports, although variations relating to protective equipment and conditioning will be present. the following is a simple guide to help you to avoid injury:

Warm-up

A warm-up is a vital part of injury prevention in every sport. It also helps to prepare you mentally and physically. Warm-ups should get the heart rate up to increase the flow of blood around the body, in preparation for more strenuous activity. It should also warm and stretch the muscles to ensure they are working to their optimum and do not sustain an injury due to being cold and inflexible.

A warm-up should consist of a minimum of 5 minutes cardio, pulse-raising exercise such as jogging, cycling, skipping etc. This should be followed by dynamic stretches. These have more recently replaced the use of static stretches. They include drills such as running with high knees, heels to bum and Cariocas, although baseball players should also concentrate on upper body warm-ups. This should be performed for a minimum of 5 minutes, up to a maximum of 20 minutes, with movements gradually becoming larger and faster. This is preferable to static stretching as it keeps the body warmer and heart rate higher, and more resembles the type of movements which are required in most sports.

Protection

Wearing the right kind of protective equipment is vital to avoiding injury in baseball. The most important position in terms of protective equipment must be the catcher. It is necessary to wear a helmet with face guard, a chest protector, throat protector, leg guards and catching mitts. The batter should also wear a helmet and batting gloves. Other protective equipment includes padded shorts and a cup.

Rest

Resting is an important part of any athletes training program! Physiological changes in the cardiovascular, respiratory, and muscular systems in our bodies, occur when we are at rest. Overtraining often results in injuries due to fatigue causing poor technique and overuse type injuries. If you feel at all unwell, tired or in pain, you should rest until better.

Training

In order to play in the higher levels of any sport, training is vitally important. Training not only the cardiovascular and muscular systems but also techniques and tactics are required to make sure the body is strong, coordinated and flexible as well as the mind is prepared and focused to name but a few.

Nutrition and Hydration

Proper nutrition is important. A bad diet will prevent you from recovering from training sessions making you more prone to injury. A balanced diet is what you should aim for:

- Carbohydrate is important for refueling muscles.
- Protein rebuilds muscles.
- If you become dehydrated then less blood will flow through muscles. The muscles will be more prone to injury.
- Vitamins and minerals are required for a number of reasons related to recovery.

A biomechanical analysis can help identify possible injury risks. Orthotic devices can help. Also, an assessment from a sports therapist or specialist can identify weak areas and possible injury risks. A course of exercises specific to your needs can give you the best chance of avoiding injury.

FOOTBALL INJURIES

It's no surprise that the most common football injuries tend to affect your lower body. That includes your hip, groin, thigh, hamstring, knee, calf, shin, ankle and foot. You might get an injury from tackling, running, shooting, twisting and turning, jumping or landing. You might also get an injury from using the same muscles repeatedly (overuse), hurting an area you've injured before if it's weak (reinjury), from foul play or colliding with your opponent. You're also more likely to become injured during a competitive match than during training sessions. Here are a few common football injuries to look out for.

Ankle Sprain

When you play football, you're often running on an uneven surface and have to change direction at a moment's notice. This means that the ligaments which stabilise your ankle joint could become overstretched, and could cause your ankle to roll inwards or outwards.

Hamstring Strain

Your hamstrings are the three large and powerful muscles at the back of your thigh. They produce a driving force during acceleration when you run. Playing football often involves quick changes of pace, going from a complete stop to quick speed in just a couple of seconds. If your hamstrings don't have enough length (from stretching) or strength, they can become quickly overloaded which could cause an injury.

To help prevent a hamstring strain, make sure to stretch them and use a foam roller regularly. A foam roller is a cylindrical device you use to massage and relieve sore and tight muscles. It can also help to work on strengthening your hamstring muscles using exercises such as deadlifts, leg curls and hamstring bridges, alongside some sport-specific speed drills.

Groin Strain

When you're on the pitch, kicking, twisting running or jumping could injure your inner thigh muscles (also known as your adductors), resulting in a groin strain. To help prevent getting a groin strain from football, be sure to stretch your inner thighs regularly and include strengthening exercises such as adductor side bridges and side lunges in your exercise routine.

Anterior Cruciate Ligament (ACL) Injury

Your ACL is a very important stabilising ligament in your knee and is most commonly injured if your lower leg stays planted while the upper part of your leg twists or moves. For example during a tackle or when landing a jump whilst moving. Whilst a full tear to your ACL would most likely need surgery, a sprain to your ACL can be managed with physiotherapy and intensive rehabilitation.

If you injure your knee and it's still painful and swollen after several days, it's important to seek the help of a physiotherapist. They can assess the extent of the damage and decide the most appropriate course of action for you.

Other possible injuries from football could include:

- Achilles tendinopathy,
- Posterior cruciate ligament (PCL) injury,
- Calf strain,
- Torn meniscus,
- Shin splints,
- Concussion,
- Quadriceps strain.

If you do sustain an injury during football, it's best to take it easy and allow your body to rest for at least a few days. Follow the steps in the PRICE and HARM graphics below for the first couple of days. If your symptoms continue, speak to a physiotherapist who may be able to help speed up your recovery. They can also give you exercises to strengthen your muscles which may prevent you getting a similar injury in the future.

Tips for Preventing Football Injuries

When it comes to any type of sport or physical activity, there are steps you can take to lower your chance of getting an injury. Here are my top tips for looking after your body when you're playing football.

- Strengthen your lower limbs

  Away from the pitch, do some lower limb strengthening exercises such as calf raises, squats, lunges and deadlifts to ensure your major muscle groups are adequately prepared to cope with the demand of a football game.

- Warm up

  Taking just a few minutes to warm up properly before football will prepare your body for exercise and reduce your risk of injury. Do some dynamic stretching (stretching whilst moving such as leg swings and knees up) alongside some jogging to increase blood flow to your muscles. Add in some ball drills involving some changing direction and speed.

- Cool down

  Spending a bit of time after the game cooling down will also help to reduce your risk of injury. Spend around 10 minutes doing some low-intensity cardiovascular exercise and stretch all your lower limbs thoroughly.

- Wear the right gear

  Protect your body by wearing the right type of clothing. It's worth getting fitted with some good boots and wearing shin guards too. If you're training outdoors, protect your skin from the sun and use a sunscreen with SPF30 and a star rating of 5.

- Eat a healthy diet

  Staying hydrated and eating the right foods will help to fuel your body during exercise and to recover afterwards.

- Get enough rest

  Be sure to get plenty of rest in between training and matches and give your body the time it needs to repair. If you're feeling any pain or are unsure if you've hurt yourself, listen to your body and take a bit of time out to recuperate. Better to miss one match than to end up injured and on the bench for the rest of the season.

RUNNING INJURIES

In an ideal runner's world, every step of every mile would be 100 percent pain-free. No aches, no twinges, no lingering soreness from yesterday's workout. The reality is that many runners constantly deal with a slight (or not so slight) disturbance—a tender foot, a tight hamstring, a whiny knee. While these nagging issues often aren't serious enough to require a time-out, they are annoying, especially when they don't let you fully enjoy your time on the roads.

Think of running pains in terms of a spectrum. At one end you have severe, full-blown injuries—call it the red zone, which includes stress fractures that require time off. The other end, where you're in top form, is the green zone. Mild, transient aches that bug you one day and disappear the next sit closer to the green end. Unfortunately, many runners get stuck in the middle—the not-quite-injured but not-quite-healthy yellow zone.

Whether you land in the red, linger in the yellow, or return to the green end of the spectrum depends largely on how you react when that first stab of pain hits, says Richard J. Price, M.D., a sports physician at Rocky Mountain Orthopedic Associates in Grand Junction, Colorado.

"Often it comes down to whether you take a little time off now or a lot of time off later," he says. You can reduce your risk of ending up in the red zone if at the first sign of an issue, you back off your mileage, reduce the intensity of your runs, start a treatment program, and develop a proactive long-term injury-prevention strategy, such as strength training, stretching, and regular foam-rolling. "Physical therapy is like homework," Price says. "None of us likes having to do it, but if you don't do it, the issue will come back."

According to Price and a team of doctors and physical therapists consulted in the following pages, there are seven injury hotspots that most frequently plague runners. If you don't get a handle on them, these issues can trap you in that nefarious yellow zone, or worse, turn into an acute injury that forces you to take a layoff. Instead, let's those keep annoying pains in check so you can move into—and, with hope, stay in—the green zone.

Runner's Knee

Patellofemoral pain syndrome (PFPS), or "runner's knee," is the irritation of the cartilage on the underside of the patella (kneecap). About 40 percent of running injuries are knee injuries. And 13 percent of runners suffered knee pain in the past year, according to 4,500 respondents to a runnersworld.com poll. PFPS typically flares up during or after long runs, after extended periods of sitting, or while descending hills and stairs.

Who's at Risk?

Anyone with biomechanical factors that put extra load on the knee is vulnerable to PFPS, says Bryan Heiderscheit, Ph.D., P.T., director of the University of Wisconsin Runners' Clinic. Risk factors include overpronation (excessive inward foot rolling) and weak quads, hips, or glutes.

Can you Run through it?

Yes, but taking extra rest days and reducing your mileage is necessary. Run every other day and only as far as you can go without pain. Some runners find that uphill running is less painful, so Heiderscheit recommends simulating hills on a treadmill. Uphill running has the added value of working your glutes. Strong gluteal muscles help control hip and thigh movement, preventing the knees from turning inward. Avoid running downhill, which can exacerbate pain. Bicycling may speed your recovery by strengthening the quads. Elliptical training and swimming are other knee-friendly activities.

Rehab it

Strengthen weak hip and glute muscles with lateral side steps, says Charlie Merrill, M.S.P.T., a physical therapist at ALTA Physical Therapy in Boulder, Colorado. Place a loop of resistance band just above your ankles or your knees. Separate your feet and bend your knees, lowering down into a slightly crouched position. While staying in this position, walk sideways 10 to 15 steps, keeping your feet straight and your upper body still. Then reverse directions. Keep your feet separated to maintain band tension. When this becomes easy, try doing this on your toes with your heels off the ground. If there's a problem in the way your kneecap tracks, athletic tape may reduce pain (Merrill demonstrates knee taping at runnersworld.com/kneetape). Post-run icing also provides relief in the early stages of this injury. Heat works best once the injury is healing and no longer in an acute stage.

Prevent a Relapse

Heiderscheit recommends shortening your stride length and landing with the knee slightly bent, which can take up to 30 percent load off the joint. Count the number of steps you take per minute and increase by five to 10 percent per minute. Keep your knee tracking correctly by strengthening your knee's support muscles like quads and glutes with exercises like lateral side steps and squats. It's also important to stretch your hip flexors.

Elite Treatment

Eventual marathon winner Meb Keflezighi was building up for the 2010 Boston Marathon when he slipped on ice and tweaked his knee. He took two weeks off, ran only every other day for the next two weeks, and then decided not to run a half marathon in March. The strategy worked: He was the second American at Boston that year, running a 2:09.

Knee Check: Process

Stop: Pain on the inside or outside of the knee immediately upon waking, which doesn't go away as the day progresses.

Caution: Twinges early in run but often dissipates or varies intermittently. Pain returns after run. Bothersome after prolonged sitting.

Run sign: Completely pain-free—even after sitting through a two-hour movie or after going on a long run with some significant incline.

Achilles Tendinitis

The Achilles tendon connects the two major calf muscles to the back of the heel. Under too much stress, the tendon tightens and becomes irritated (tendinitis). It makes up 11 percent of all running injuries; eight percent of runnersworld.com poll respondents dealt with it this past year.

Who's at Risk?

Runners who dramatically increase training (especially hills and speedwork) and have tight, weak calves are vulnerable.

Can you Run through it?

"If you have any pain during or after running, stop," says Amol Saxena, D.P.M., a sports podiatrist in Palo Alto, Calif. "This is not an injury to run through."

If you catch a minor strain early, a few days off might be sufficient healing time. If you keep running as usual, you could develop a serious case that may take six months to go away.

Rehab it

Five times a day, apply ice. Strengthen the calves with eccentric heel drops: Stand with the balls of your feet on a step. Rise up on both feet. Once up, take your stronger foot off the step. Lower down on your injured foot, dropping your heel below the step. Rise back up, return your other foot to the step. Do 20 reps. Pool-run, use an elliptical machine, and swim, but avoid cycling unless it's not painful.

Prevent a Relapse

Strong calves protect your Achilles from flare-ups, Dr. Price says, so do heel drops daily. Avoid aggressive calf stretching and wearing flip-flops and high heels, all of which can irritate the Achilles.

Elite Treatment

Shannon Rowbury, 1500-meter bronze medalist (2009 World Championships), wears compression socks for hard workouts to relieve Achilles tightness.

"It's made a huge difference," she says.

Ankle Alert: Process

You experience severe pain and swelling above your heel—even when not running. Standing up on your toes causes pain.

Caution: There is a dull pain around your heel at the end of your run that continues to linger afterward, but eventually goes away when iced.

Run sign: You feel no pain when pinching the tendon, starting at the heel and working your way up your leg, toward your calf.

Hamstring Issues

The muscles that run down the back of our thighs bend our knees, extend our legs, drive us up hills, and power finish-line kicks. So when our hamstrings are too tight or weak to perform well, we notice it. Seven percent of poll respondents say their hamstrings have bugged them this past year.

Who's at Risk?

Hamstring issues usually arise because these muscles are weak—often from being too long or too short. Counterintuitive as it might seem, very flexible people are prone to hamstring problems because their overly stretched-out muscles are more vulnerable to damage. On the flip side, people who can barely touch their toes or who sit for long periods of time are also at risk. Tight, short muscles are under greater tension. Another factor is muscle imbalance: Many runners' quadriceps overpower their hamstrings, which sets them up for injury.

Can you Run through it?

If the pain comes on suddenly and strong and the area bruises, you may have a true pull and you'll need extended rest—months—before you can run again. If it's a less severe, chronic overuse injury, you can usually run, but it'll take some time before you're back in the green zone. "Hamstring issues stink," Price says. "It takes a long time to heal them." Running a slow, easy pace is usually less bothersome than attempting intervals or hill repeats. Bicycling, pool running, and swimming are good alternative activities.

Rehab it

Strengthen your hamstrings with one-legged hamstring curls (raise the bar with both legs, then slowly lower it one leg at a time) and one-legged deadlifts. Use a foam roller to alleviate tightness before and after a run, Merrill says. In chronic cases, active release technique (ART) and deep-tissue massage may be necessary.

Prevent a Relapse

Stay strong with bridges: Lie on your back with your feet on a chair or exercise ball. Raise your hips, then lift one leg into the air. Slowly lower your hips back down to the floor, using the supporting leg. Return that leg to the ball. Repeat with the other leg. Also, compression tights during or after running can aid blood flow.

Elite Treatment

When U.S. champion miler David Torrence felt his hamstring tighten up, he took the next day off and went to his chiropractor.

"My pelvis was misaligned, causing my hamstring to do extra work," he says. "I took it easy for a few days, iced the hamstring four times throughout the day, and was improved within a week."

Hamstring Signs: Process

Stop: If you experience sharp, sudden, strong pain and possibly even a snap or pop sound while running. The area is bruised.

Caution: The presence of a stubborn chronic achiness and tightness that forces you to slow your pace and shorten your stride.

Run sign: If you are pain-free even while climbing hills and doing speed work, and your hamstring is unaffected by extended periods of sitting.

Plantar Fasciitis

It's not shocking that about 15 percent of all running injuries strike the foot—with each step, our feet absorb a force several times our body weight. Plantar fasciitis, small tears or inflammation of the tendons and ligaments that run from your heel to your toes, is usually the top foot complaint among runners—10 percent of runnersworld.com poll respondents struggled with it this past year. The pain, which typically feels like a dull ache or bruise along your arch or on the bottom of your heel, is usually worse first thing in the morning.

Who's at Risk?

Runners with very high or very low arches are vulnerable, Saxena says, because both foot types cause the plantar fascia to be stretched away from the heel bone. Other causes are extreme pronation (foot rolls inward excessively) or supination (foot rolls outward excessively) and increasing your mileage too quickly. Long periods of standing, especially on hard floors without supportive footwear, may exacerbate the problem. Tight hip flexors, weak core muscles, and a history of lower back pain can also contribute.

"Back issues and core weakness can lead to subtle changes in your stride that you'll feel in the feet," Merrill says.

Can you Run through it?

Plantar fasciitis is one of the most notoriously nagging injuries, and running through it, while possible, can delay healing. Recovery time can range from three months to a year, but six months is fairly typical, Saxena says. In chronic cases, a complete break from running is usually best. Pool running and swimming keep pressure off your feet. Cycling or using an elliptical can help you maintain fitness, but only if you can do those activities without pain. Wearing a Strassburg sock while you relax keeps your arch from tightening up.

Rehab it

Roll your foot over a frozen water bottle for five minutes at a time, five times a day, Saxena says. To stretch your plantar fascia, sit with one leg crossed over the other so that your right ankle rests on your left knee. Grab the end of your right foot at the toes and gently pull back. Because calf tightness can be a factor, Merrill also recommends using a foam roller to loosen them up. He also stresses the importance of doing core work (planks, back extensions).

"When I see someone who has had plantar pain for years, they're almost always missing core strength," Merrill says. "Sometimes all they need is some core work and their heel gets better. A stable core reduces stress on the spine and stops pain transference to the foot."

Prevent a Relapse

Make sure your shoes fit your foot type by getting an analysis at a running shoe store or from a podiatrist or physical therapist, says Saxena. A custom orthotic may even help. Stretch and massage the plantar fascia several times a day. In the morning, hang your feet over the edge of the bed and roll your ankles. Do core work at least twice a week.

Elite Treatment

Magdalena Lewy Boulet, a 2:26 marathoner, struggled with plantar fasciitis in 2007 that became so severe she contemplated ending her career.

"I got on a rehab routine that included active-isolated stretching, and it cured me," she says. "Now it's part of my maintenance routine. I do it for about 15 minutes twice a day."

Foot Wary: Process

Stop: Ongoing, ever-present arch pain and tenderness that doesn't seem to fade even once you've warmed up on a run.

Caution: If you experience any pain when you step out of bed, get up after sitting for a long time, or during the first few minutes of a run.

Run sign: When you are pain-free all day, including your first steps in the morning. Walking barefoot on hard surfaces isn't an issue.

Shin Splints

"Shin splints" refers to medial tibial stress syndrome, an achy pain that results when small tears occur in the muscles around your tibia (shin bone). This makes up about 15 percent of running injuries; 10 percent of runnersworld.com respondents poll had shinsplints in the past year.

Who's at Risk?

Shinsplints are common among new runners and those returning after an extended layoff. They're a sign that you've done too much, too quickly, Dr. Price says. Shinsplints strike runners wearing the wrong shoe or a pair with too many miles, and those with high arches or flat feet.

Can you Run through it?

When the first twinges of pain strike, back off your running to a comfortable level for a few days to a week, then slowly up your mileage using the 10 percent rule (no more than 10 percent increase per week). Bike, pool run, and swim.

Rehab it

Rest, ice, and ibuprofen can ease the pain. Though conventional wisdom has preached calf stretching as a way to rehabilitate shinsplints, there's little evidence that helps, Price says. Taping the shin with Kinesio Tex tape can relieve pain and speed healing. Wearing an air cast ankle brace throughout the day—even while running—can speed recovery. These braces stabilize the ankle so the shin muscles don't have to work so hard to support your leg, Saxena says.

Prevent a Relapse

The easiest and best way to avoid shinsplints is to increase mileage gradually. Saxena also says to make sure you are in an appropriate shoe. Beginners, especially, can benefit from the professional help at a specialty running shop. If you have high arches, you may need a cushioned shoe. Or if you have flat feet, a rigid shoe might be the solution, he says.

Elite Treatment

Once or twice a month, miler David Torrence jumps in a game of pickup basketball or soccer.

"The lateral movement uses your muscles differently than running in one direction," he says. "It's helped me manage my shinsplints."

Shin Signs: Process

Stop: Tenderness down the leg—especially if you hop on it. If even walking (not just running) hurts, it could be a fracture.

Caution: You experience a tight, aching pain when running—but the pain goes away when you stop. Hopping isn't painful.

Run sign: When you are completely pain-free while running—even long after you stop applying ice after runs and taping your shins.

Iliotibial Band Syndrome (ITBS)

The iliotibial (IT) band lies along the outside of the thigh from the hip to the knee. When you run, your knee flexes and extends, which causes the IT band to rub on the side of the femur. This can cause irritation if you take up your mileage too quickly, especially if you're doing a lot of track work or downhill running. ITBS makes up 12 percent of all running injuries; 14 percent of poll respondents experienced this in the past year.

Who's at Risk?

Runners who develop ITBS may overpronate, have a leg-length discrepancy, or suffer from weak hip abductor and gluteal muscles.

"If your hip motion is not well controlled, then your IT band gets stretched with your running stride, and that can irritate it," Heiderscheit says.

Can you Run Through It?

ITBS is known as a stubborn, nagging injury. Take a rest day or two and back off your mileage for a week, and you could avoid a full-blown flare-up, Dr. Price says. If you ignore the first symptoms and continue training at your usual mileage and intensity, you can exacerbate it.

Rehab It

Strengthen the hip abductors with lateral side steps, side leg lifts, and one-legged squats. Use a foam roller before and after you run: Rest the outside of your thigh on top of the roller, and roll your IT band from your knee to your hip. Hiking and bicycling can aggravate ITBS. Instead, swim, pool-run, and use an elliptical trainer.

Prevent a Relapse

Continue exercises and foam-rolling. Change directions every few laps while on a track, and limit how often you do hilly routes, Heiderscheit says. IT band issues often get better if you can learn to shorten your stride so that your weight centers on the front of the heel or the midfoot as you land.

"A five to 10 percent difference in your stride length can make a huge difference," Heiderscheit says.

Elite Treatment

Two-time Olympian (5000 meters) Bolota Asmerom, of Oakland, Calif., dealt with ITBS when he took up his training to 70 miles a week in 1999.

"I got relief through massage, strength, and flexibility work," he says. "I've stayed injury-free since then because I take care of every ache with massage and ice. I also try to avoid doing too much track running."

Thigh Anxiety: Process

Stop: If you experience pain on the outside of the knee that radiates up and down your leg when just walking down a hill or stairs.

Caution: When twinges on the outside of the knee appear within 10 minutes of beginning a run, but disappear during a walk break.

Run sign: When your outer knee and thigh are completely pain-free—even after running a particularly hilly route or circling a track.

Stress Fracture

Unlike an acute fracture that happens as the result of a slip or fall, stress fractures develop as a result of cumulative strain on the bone. Runners most often have stress fractures in their tibias (shin), metatarsals (feet), or calcaneus (heels). They are one of the most serious of all running injuries; almost six percent of poll respondents had one in the past year.

Who's at Risk?

Runners who overtrain. Bones need downtime to rebuild after a workout. If you increase the duration, intensity, or frequency of your running too soon, your bones can't repair themselves fast enough to keep up. Stress fractures are more common in women than men, usually due to nutritional deficits, low estrogen levels, and inadequate calorie intake. Luckily, weight-bearing exercise like running is protective, which means experience is on your side. "The longer you've been running, the lower your risk is," Dr. Price says.

Can you Run Through It?

In a word: no. Expect to take eight to 16 weeks off from running. The amount of rest you'll need depends on the severity of the fracture and its location. Weight-bearing bones like those in the foot heal slower than those in the shin, for example. And if you ran through the pain for a while before you realized you had a fracture, your recovery could take longer, Merrill says. Avoid all impact exercise and instead, pool-run and swim.

Rehab It

Listen-well-to your body.

"Once you can walk without any pain, you can try a bit of jogging," Dr. Price says. "But you have to back off if there is lingering pain. It's crucial that you build your mileage slowly-start with just a few minutes."

Prevent a Relapse

Improve bone density with weight training, and make sure you're getting enough calories and nutrients. Contrary to popular belief, running surfaces don't seem to make a difference.

"It makes sense that running on soft surfaces like grass would be better than roads, but studies have not borne that out," Price says.

Elite Treatment

Some people with stress fractures can maintain fitness with pool running.

"When Deena Kastor suffered a broken bone in her foot during the 2008 Olympic Marathon, she had to take six weeks off," Price says. "Daily pool running kept her strong."

After making a recovery, she ran a 2:28 Chicago Marathon in 2009.

Bone Scan: Process

Stop: If pain continues to build as you run-but it doesn't just hurt when you run. Even just being on your feet is uncomfortable.

Caution: Sorry, there's no middle ground here. With this injury, you are either in the red and should be shut down, or in the green zone and good to go.

Run sign: When you're pain-free throughout a run with absolutely no lingering pain afterward-even when you've been on your feet all day.

SWIMMING INJURIES

Recent trends have shown a sharp increase in youth sports participation and athletic activities, including swimming. With the increase in participation, there has been a concomitant rise in the number of sports-related injuries. A majority of these injuries are due to overuse as athletes are frequently competing in multiple sports or in year-round competition and training. Additionally, increasingly higher demands are put upon these young athletes, increasing their likelihood of sustaining a season-compromising and possibly career-ending injury.

With overuse comes fatigue and lapses in appropriate swimming technique. Often swimmers demonstrate tremendous flexibility or joint laxity, which can be normal, but when swimmers repetitively move through an inappropriate range of motion due to poor technique, slight injuries and micro-trauma can cause shoulders, low backs and knees to become painful.

Swimmers' Shoulder

The shoulder is the joint most commonly affected by swimming injuries or overuse. Shoulder injuries may include rotator cuff impingement (pressure on the rotator cuff as the hand is 'catching' water at the beginning of the pull), biceps tendinitis (painful inflammation of the bicep tendon) and shoulder instability (in which structures that surround the shoulder joint do not work to maintain the ball within its socket). Each of these conditions can result from fatigue and weakness of the rotator cuff and muscles surrounding the shoulder blade.

Low back Pain

Due to the increased amount of time that swimmers spend with their backs in a hyper-extended position, as well as their tendency to have higher than average flexibility in their joints and decreased core strength, it is common for elite level swimmers to complain of low back pain resulting from lumbar disc disease or spondylosis.

Breaststrokers' Knee

Knee injuries that involve the tendons and ligaments along the inside of the knee (breaststrokers' knee) are common. These kinds of injuries, as well as other knee and hip pain in swimmers, are often caused by core weakness, hyper-mobility and other muscle imbalances.

Treatment of Common Swimming Injuries

Common treatment protocols for shoulder, low back and knee pain often include components of stretching and strengthening the shoulder complex, core stabilization, and correcting muscle imbalances. The exercises depicted here are some examples of exercises that can be done to prevent excess laxity in the shoulder complex, as well as to improve core and shoulder stability.

Additionally, should the athlete experience pain with swimming that persists, they should see a doctor, physical therapist, or athletic trainer for a full diagnostic work-up and care plan.

Swimming Exercises

Sleeper Stretch

Lay on your side with your head supported, your bottom arm perpendicular to your body, and your elbow bent to 90 degrees. With your top hand, gently push your forearm toward the table until you feel a slight stretch or resistance by your shoulder blade. Hold 30 seconds. Repeat 3 times.

External Rotation

Lay on your side with your head supported. Place a towel roll under your elbow. Start with your hand near your belly button and raise until your forearm is parallel with the ground (as pictured). Start without weight and complete 20 repetitions 2 times.

Plank

Start on your elbows and toes. Keep your back flat by pulling your belly button toward your spine and pushing your tailbone towards your heels. Keep your shoulder blades rounded, without pinching them together and hold 30 seconds. Repeat 3 times.

Double knee-to-chest Stretch

Lie on the floor with your back relaxed and straight. Pull both knees toward your chest until you feel a stretch in your lower back. Do not bounce. Hold 5 seconds. Repeat 5 times.

Hamstring Stretch

Keep your chest up and maintain a curvature in your lower back as you lean forward. Do not allow the knee on the leg being stretched to bend up. Hold 30 seconds. Repeat 3 times. Seated hamstring stretch can be done on the floor. Sit with one knee bent and the bottom of your foot against the inside of the opposite thigh.

Hamstring Curls

Start with both feet on a stability ball, with hips lifted. Keeping your core and abs tight, draw your heels toward you, keeping your hips elevated (as pictured). Complete 20 repetitions 2 times.

RACQUET INJURIES

Racquet sports (tennis, racquetball, squash, badminton, and paddle tennis) are sports of speed and agility and involve athletes of all ages. As in many sports, the risk of injury increases with age due to the style of play, contact forces, and size of athletes. However, the risk of injuries can be reduced.

The following is information from the American Academy of Pediatrics (AAP) about how to choose a racquet and prevent racquet sports injuries. Also included is an overview of common injuries and treatment.

Injury Prevention and Safety Tips

- Sports physical exam: Athletes should have a preparticipation physical evaluation (PPE) to make sure they are ready to safely begin the sport. The best time for a PPE is about 4 to 6 weeks before the beginning of the season. Athletes also should see their doctors for routine checkups.
- Fitness: Athletes should maintain a good fitness level during the season and off-season. Preseason training should allow time for general conditioning and sportspecific conditioning. Also important are proper warmup and cool-down exercises.
- Technique: Athletes should learn and practice safe techniques for performing the skills that are integral to their sport. Examples of poor technique include not fully extending the elbow on forehands or backhands, hitting the ball too late, and serving behind one's head. Athletes should work with coaches and athletic trainers on achieving proper technique.
- Training: A good rule of thumb is not to increase training by more than 10% per week. That means if an athlete is playing 10 hours per week, the following week could be 11 hours not 20 hours.
- Exercises: Some young athletes are weak in their shoulder, trunk, or leg muscles. It is wise to do appropriate strengthening exercises for these muscle groups. Others are inflexible in the hamstrings, hips, or shoulders and need appropriate stretching exercises. A certified strength and conditioning coach or athletic trainer can demonstrate appropriate exercises.
- Equipment: Safety gear includes,
    - Protective eyewear: Glasses or goggles should be made with polycarbonate or a similar material. The material should conform to the standards of the American Society for Testing and Materials (ASTM).
    - Sun protection (ie, sunscreen, lip balm with sunblock) when outdoors
- Environment: Athletes used to playing on a soft surface (clay or grass) should gradually change to a hard surface. For example, 10 hours per week on soft surface; 1 hour per week on hard surface. Also, extra balls on the playing surface should be cleared away so that no one steps on them.

CLIMBING INJURIES

While scrapes and bruises are synonymous with climbing, just like any other sport, intense physical activity increases your susceptibility to injury. Ignoring an injury and pushing through the pain will only worsen your condition. Luckily, you can mitigate climbing injuries with proper training practices and good habits.

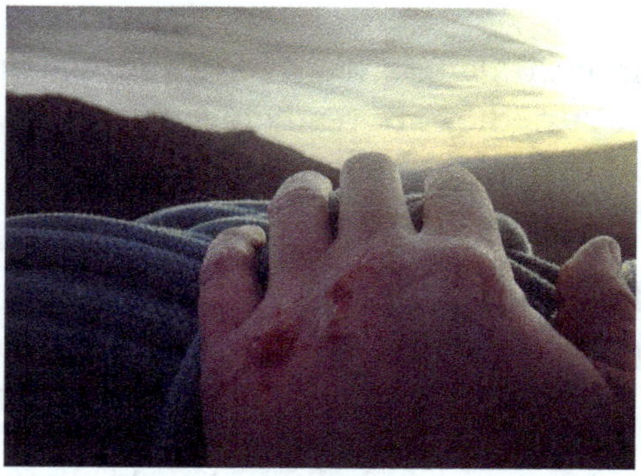

Finger Pulley Tears

Finger pulley tears are one of the most common climbing injuries and they're pretty unique to the sport. A finger pulley tear results from overloading a finger tendon with your body weight, likely resulting from a dynamic move or crimping.

These injuries often occur when utilising one or two fingers in a pocket or gripping a small hold with the tips of your fingers. Often, you will hear and feel an actual pop. Pain immediately follows and swelling will develop shortly afterwards.

Finger pulleys, or annular pulleys keep the tendon that flexes the finger from "bow-stringing" away from the finger bone. They're ofern refered to by the number, A1, A2, etc. With an A2 being one of the most common injuries of this type.

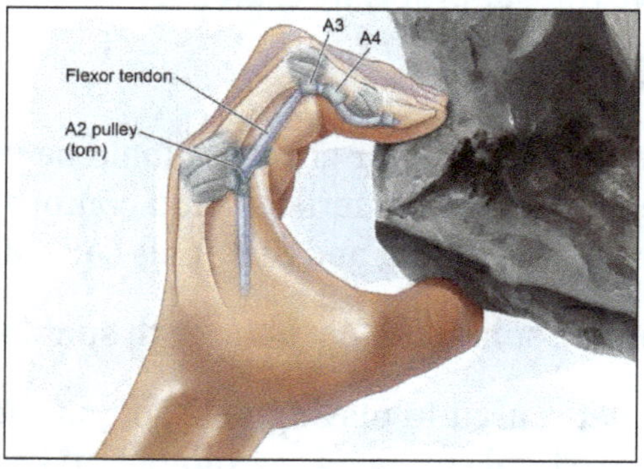

Finger pulley tears are frustrating because they take a while to heal. Applying ice and taking an anti-inflammatory is the first step to healing a finger pulley injury.

You're going to need to take time off climbing until your fingers have healed. When easing back into climbing, stick to big jugs and other holds that avoid putting direct pressure on the injured finger(s). Taping these fingers while climbing during the healing process is an effective way to prevent worsening the injury.

Prevention: The best way to prevent finger pulley tears is to build up your finger strength slowly. Although your forearms might be strong enough to crimp on tiny 5.12 holds, your fingers might not yet have the strength. It takes more time to build strength in your tendons.

Hang boarding is a great way to build finger strength, but start slow, and take it easy. If you're a beginner, give the hang board a miss and focus on climbing more at a moderate grade. Finger pulley tears can result in major training setbacks. Utilise every ounce of prevention.

Shoulder Subluxation

Climbers who boulder or make large, overhead moves are especially susceptible to shoulder subluxation, which is a partial dislocation of the shoulder.

It happens as result of extending the shoulder's ball joint too far forward. You will feel a sharp pain in the back of your shoulder and need to stop climbing immediately, as continued movement could result in a full dislocation.

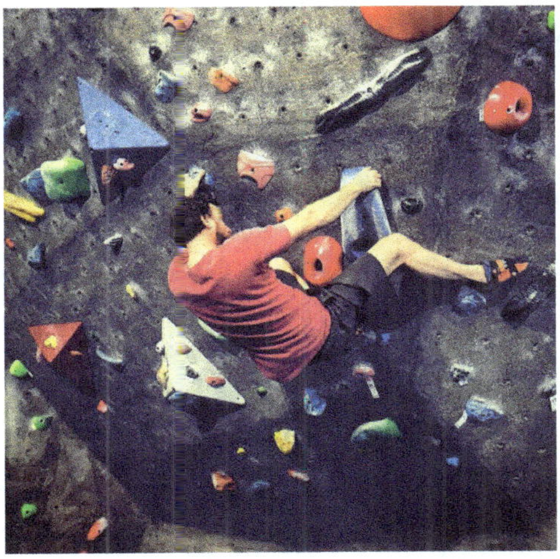

Recovery will require physical therapy and medical care. Stretching and conditioning routines will help you regain full strength and range of movement.

Prevention: Stretching to warm up the shoulders is a great way to prevent subluxations. Yoga is an especially effective way to build shoulder strength.

Be sure to ease into difficult movements. Start on easy grades and work your way up, backing off if you ever start to feel any kind of discomfort. Warming up and cooling down on the wall is a good way to help prevent shoulder injuries.

Rotator Cuff Tears

A rotator cuff tear is another serious shoulder injury. As opposed to dislocation, it's also possible to tear the muscles in your shoulder.

Climbing is a unique sport in that we spend much of the time with our arms extended above our shoulders, which puts stress on the tendons. Pain and aching in your upper arms and shoulders when you lift your arms above your head signifies a minor tear. You may also experience some weakness and numbness.

Ice and rest are the best treatments for minor tears. More serious tears could require medical attention, so after any injury it's important to consult a doctor. Physical therapy may also be helpful during the healing process to ensure that your shoulders regain their full range of motion.

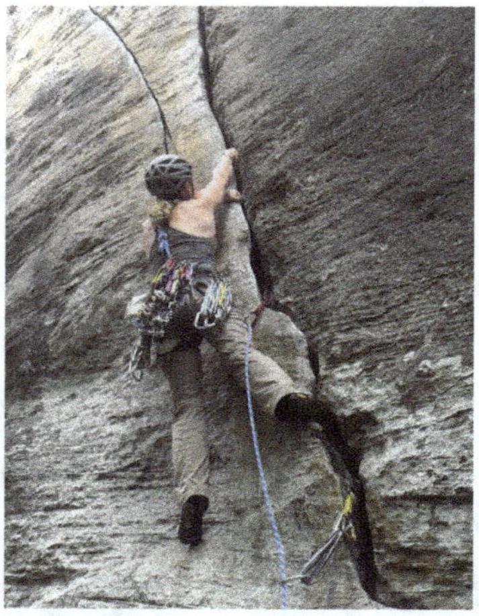

Prevention: As with most shoulder injuries, stretching is a great way to prevent rotator cuff tears. Increase the strength in your shoulders by implementing cable machine exercises that involve internal and external rotations. Lateral shoulder flys with weights is another great exercise to help build shoulder strength.

Tendonitis

The general definition of tendonitis is inflammation or irritation of a tendon.

The most common symptom is a dull aching pain, often accompanied by swelling. Tendons are the cords that attach muscle to bone. In climbers, tendonitis most often occurs in the shoulders, elbows and forearms. Other names for tendonitis:

- Tennis elbow
- Jumper's knee
- Pitcher's shoulder

Although these names refer to other sports associated with the condition, you can link climbing to tendonitis in any part of the body.

Tendonitis is more of a chronic condition than the result of immediate trauma and can worsen over time. It is caused by constantly pulling on the same muscles and stems from repetitive movements. It's important to take tendonitis seriously so that it doesn't develop into a tendon rupture - a much more serious injury that could require surgery. Treating tendonitis means taking a break from climbing, resting, and applying ice.

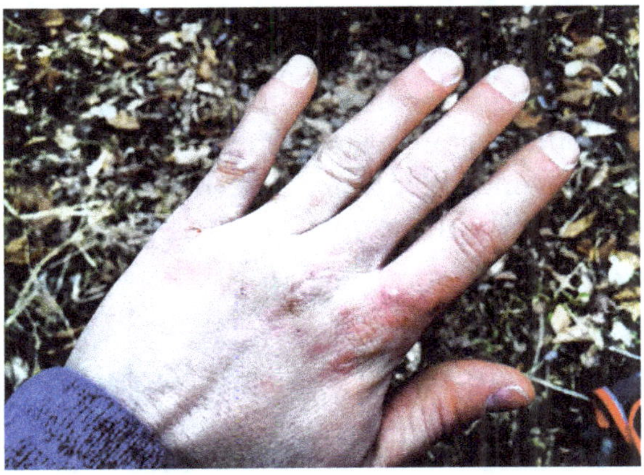

Prevention: Again stretching and conditioning are key here. Extensor and flexor exercises on a cable machine are especially helpful. Start with a little weight and add more over time to build strength before you hit the wall.

Do exercises that help build grip and forearm strength, as well. A hang board can be a helpful tool in this case as well, but again you need to be careful to start slowly.

Trigger Finger Syndrome

Trigger finger syndrome is a condition in which your fingers lock up when you bend them. You might notice a popping sound or clicking sound and some stiffness. In this situation, a cyst has actually formed inside the flexor tendons in your finger, leaving you with limited gripping potential, which can be frustrating while climbing, although not typically painful.

Symptoms tend to start out mild but progress over time. The only real treatment is rest, anti-inflammatories, and in some cases, acupuncture can be effective.

Prevention: The best way to prevent trigger finger syndrome is to mix up your climbing style and training routine.

If you boulder one day, lead climb the next day, do top rope laps on moderate routes the third day, and be sure to take rest days. Gentle finger exercises and massage can also reduce the probability of occurrence.

Cracked Feet

While those super tight climbing shoes help you climb hard, they can wreak havoc on your feet. Dryness and trauma associated with crack climbing or heel hooking can result in cracked feet - most commonly at the point of the heel. This makes putting on your climbing shoes the next day extremely painful. While not life threatening, it can sure cramp your style, so it's important to take preventative measures.

Prevention: Keep your feet soft and supple with a daily lotion application, before and after you climb. In the event of a cracked sole or heel, apply a healing salve and switch up your climbing style.

It's also important to avoid overexposure to chemicals, wet conditions, and extreme cold, all of which can attribute to cracked feet. Stay off those cracks and overhangs until your feet heal - go seek out some killer slab routes instead or set your sights on a long, moderate multi-pitch route in the meantime.

Abrasions

While bruises and abrasions are simply a part of climbing, when cracks leave your hands absolutely wrecked and covered in wounds which climbers affectionately call 'gobies', it might be time to think about taking measures to mitigate the occurrence or severity of these injuries.

Abrasions result from scraping your skin against rock. Sharp rock is an especially renowned abrasion culprit. Although not life threatening, these injuries take time to heal, and preventative measures go a long way.

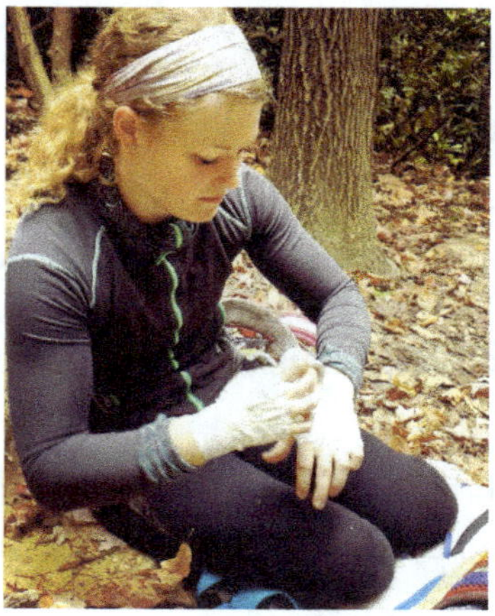

Prevention: When it comes to your hands, tape gloves are your best bet at prevention. Many climbing apparel companies also sell climbing specific gloves for crack climbers.

Yoga is a great addition to any climbing training regime as it helps you stretch and strengthens many important muscles and builds overall flexibility.

References

- Five-common-basketball-injuries, post: muellersportsmed.com, Retrieved 25 April, 2019
- Baseball-injuries, sports-specific, sport-injuries: sportsinjuryclinic.net, Retrieved 26 May, 2019
- Common-football-injuries, ourviews, newsroom: bupa.co.uk, Retrieved 27 June, 2019
- How-to-prevent-and-treat-common-running-injuries, running: active.com, Retrieved 28 July, 2019
- Common-swimming-injuries-and-how-to-treat-them: mercyhealthsystem.org, Retrieved 29 August, 2019
- Racquet-Sports, Pages, sports, healthy-living, English: healthychildren.org, Retrieved 30 January, 2019
- Common-climbing-injuries-and-prevention: theclimbingguy.com, Retrieved 1 February, 2019

Sports Nutrition

CHAPTER 4

The study and practice of implementing appropriate diet and nutrition to improve the athletic performance of a person is known as sports nutrition. It studies the type and quantity of fluids and food taken by an athlete. The topics elaborated in this chapter will help in gaining a better perspective about sports nutrition as well as the different types of sports drinks which fall under it.

NUTRITION FOR SPORTS PERSONS

Diet should be optimal in both quality and quantity of food, in order to replenish your energy reserves and avoid fatigue or inadequate nutrition. A good diet will help your body perform at its best.

Specific Needs of Athletes

- Carbohydrates

  Carbohydrates are the best fuel source to provide power for your working muscles. Eating enough carbohydrate before, during and after exercise helps to maintain energy levels, delay fatigue during exercise and support a more rapid recovery. With carbohydrate or "carbs" as the main fuel source, you can maintain your activity for a longer period. Carbohydrate foods should make up more than half your total energy intake. If you are involved in heavy daily exercise, your carbohydrate needs will be even higher and you should make sure you eat enough carbohydrate to meet your increased daily requirements.

- Proteins

  Proteins are the building blocks of your body's muscles and tissues. Most athletes need only slightly more protein than non-athletes. You will usually meet your increased requirements through increased food intake. It is unlikely that you'll need protein supplements. If you are involved in aesthetic (e.g. gymnastics), weight restriction (e.g. light weight rowing) or endurance sports (e.g. marathon running), you may have higher protein requirements. Foods like meats, legumes and dairy products are good sources of protein.

- Fats

  Fat is important in the athlete's diet as it provides energy, fat-soluble vitamins and essential fatty acids. However, fat should be eaten in moderation. A low-fat diet is a good approach for everyone – athlete and non-athlete alike. Choose "good" fats such as polyunsaturated and monounsaturated fats which are found in fish, nuts, seeds, canola and olive oils and avocados.

- Vitamins and Minerals

  Vitamins and Minerals are the "spark plugs" of physical activity. Some help your body use the energy from carbohydrate, protein and fat. Others help your muscles relax and contract. If you follow a balanced diet, you will generally take in enough essential vitamins and minerals. However, if you are trying to lose weight, you may have low levels of some vitamins and minerals in your diet. Despite the best intentions, some busy people don't follow a balanced diet, so watch your intake of iron, calcium and zinc, which are especially important for physically active people.

Iron is part of haemoglobin, the part of red blood cells that carries oxygen to your body cells. Oxygen is essential for creating energy in your muscle cells. An iron shortfall, even if it's small, can affect your physical performance. Female athletes are more prone to low iron levels, as iron is lost through menstruation. Iron from foods occurs in two forms – "haem" iron found in animal foods and "non-haem" iron found in plant foods. Haem iron is readily absorbed by our bodies. In contrast, non-haem iron is poorly absorbed. If you are a vegetarian or eat mainly plant-based foods, you can increase the absorption of iron by adding a vitamin-C rich food (e.g. citrus fruits and juices, kiwi fruit, red capsicum etc) to your meals. For a further boost in iron levels, eat iron-fortified foods (e.g. breakfast cereal). The recommended dietary intake for iron is 7mg/day for adult men and 12-16mg/day for adult women.

Iron Counter

Which food?	How much iron (mg)?
Haem iron	
90g lamb liver	8.6
6 oysters	3.5
100g lean beef	2.2
120g fish (non specified type)	1.1
100g chicken breast	0.7
Non-haem iron sources	
30g bran flakes	5.4
½ cup canned chickpeas	1.6
½ cup spinach	0.6
10 macadamia nuts	0.4

- Calcium

  Calcium combined with weight-bearing activity helps to increase bone density plus build and maintain strong bones. Adults need a daily intake of 800mg calcium, and the simplest way to meet your requirements is to eat plenty of dairy products. If you are watching your weight, choose low fat dairy products which will still give you a calcium boost. Dairy foods are a good source of carbohydrates as well.

Calcium Counter

Which food? How much calcium (mg)?	How much calcium (mg)?
200g tub yogurt, reduced fat	340
2 slices (40g) cheddar cheese, reduced fat	310
100g (1/4 cup) small can pink salmon canned in brine (with bones)	280
250mL (1 glass) milk (low fat / skim)	310
¼ cup mozzarella cheese	260
1 cup vanilla ice cream	150
¼ cup almonds	70
½ cup baked beans, canned in tomato sauce	50

Magnesium is found in dried fruit, nuts and chocolate. It plays a role in energy reactions, protein production and muscle contraction.

How can you get enough carbohydrate?

Carbohydrate foods include breads, breakfast cereals, rice, pasta, fruit, vegetables and legumes (dried beans and peas). There are smaller amounts of carbohydrate in dairy products like milk and yogurt and foods with added sugars.

Carbohydrates are important to maintain blood-glucose levels during exercise and to replace muscle glycogen. Recommendations for athletes range from 6 to 10g/kg body weight per day. The amount required depends on your total daily energy expenditure, the type of sport/exercise you perform, your gender and the environmental conditions. To calculate your total daily requirement, multiply the amount of carbohydrate you require (6-10g/kg per day) by your body weight. A sports dietitian can help you determine your individual needs.

Your body's carbohydrate stores are very small and need regular replenishing, generally every 4 to 5 hours (especially if you exercise daily or twice daily). Follow these strategies to achieve a high-carbohydrate intake:

- High-carbohydrate foods should be the number one priority in your meals and snacks and should take up most of the room on your plate.

- Remember, vegetables and salads are good sources of vitamins, minerals and fibre, but they don't contribute large amounts of carbohydrate. Make sure you include pasta, rice, potatoes or legumes with your main meals.
- If you have very high carbohydrate needs, a sports dietitian can help you plan your diet to ensure you meet your requirements.

Carbohydrate Counter

Which food?	How much carbohydrate (g)?
700mL sports drink (average)	50
¾ cup boiled rice	40
1 cup cooked pasta	36
1 x 200g tub reduced fat yogurt	34
2 slices wholemeal bread	26
2.5 wheat flake breakfast biscuits	25
1 medium banana	22
1 medium potato boiled	18
1 Tbsp jam	18
1 cup cooked cous cous	15
½ cup baked beans in tomato sauce	15
250mL milk	12

Glycaemic Index

We used to think of carbohydrate foods as 'simple' or 'complex'. Foods high in sugars were considered 'simple' carbohydrates, as it was assumed they would be digested quickly and cause a rapid rise in blood glucose levels. 'Complex' carbohydrates (starches), on the other hand were thought to give a slow gradual rise in blood glucose levels. However, now a carbohydrate can be classified by its "glycaemic index" (GI). As an athlete, you can use knowledge about the carbohydrate content of foods, as well as the GI of such foods, to help optimise your performance.

The GI is a ranking of carbohydrate foods, based on their effect on our blood glucose (or blood sugar) levels. The GI ranks foods from 0–100. The higher the GI value, the greater the blood sugar response. So, low GI foods raise blood sugar levels just a little, medium GI foods raise blood sugar levels moderately, and high GI foods raise blood sugar levels quite high.

The ranking of GI foods is as follows:

- Low GI foods - less than 55
- Medium GI foods - 55 to 70
- High GI foods - more than 70

GI before Exercise

A low GI meal before exercise may help your performance. It does this by providing a sustained release of carbohydrate for your working muscles. However, as well as GI, it is important to consider other characteristics of your food such as the total carbohydrate content, nutritional value, practicality, cost, taste and how comfortable you feel exercising shortly after eating that particular food. It's best to experiment with different foods before your training sessions and not try anything new just before an important sporting event.

GI During Exercise

Eating carbohydrate during exercise, especially prolonged, intense exercise, will provide extra fuel for your working muscles and can improve performance. Moderate to high GI foods are the best choice for this type of exercise, as they act fairly quickly to raise blood glucose levels and provide your muscles with a readily available source of energy.

GI and Recovery

High GI foods provide a rapid supply of glucose to your blood and can replace your muscle glycogen stores. It is important to rebuild your glycogen stores so that you have plenty of energy for your next exercise session, particularly if your recovery time is less than eight hours. Drinking a sports drink immediately after exercise is a great way to refuel and they help replace fluids at the same time. Other examples of high GI foods include honey on a bagel, a banana sandwich, watermelon or some breakfast bars.

FLUID BALANCE

Competitive and recreational exercisers alike may drink before, during and/or after exercise. Their reasons for drinking can be wide ranging, for example, to minimise dehydration, to provide a substrate or to refresh the mouth. However, while it is also common for solid food to be consumed before and after exercise, it is much less common for solid food to be consumed during exercise, with the exception perhaps of ultra-endurance exercise.

The decision of whether to eat and/or drink or do neither during exercise will be made based upon whether the exerciser wants to do so for comfort reasons, for hydration reasons or for substrate consumption. If substrate provision is the main aim, then solid food may be as effective as liquid 'food' provided that both can be equally well tolerated. Significant amounts of carbohydrate can be provided by a relatively concentrated drink. If, however, hydration is the aim, then it is unlikely that solid food can provide the quantities of water desired. Therefore drinks play an important role in the diet of exercisers who need to pay attention to their hydration.

Sweat Loss in Exercise

Body mass changes, rather than any measure of body water change, is typically used in research studies (and applied practice) to quantify a change in hydration status. In order to ascertain the significance of these findings, it is necessary to have an understanding of the extent of body mass reductions, largely due to water loss, that an individual may experience.

Typically, maximum sweat rates are in the order of 2–3 litres per hour. Therefore, body mass reductions of up to 2–3% could feasibly occur in many exercise situations and reductions of this magnitude, and more, are reported in the scientific literature. However, it is important to remember that there is a large inter-individual variation in sweating even when the same or similar exercise is carried out in the same conditions or when individuals are exposed to the same heat stress. For example, the study of football (soccer) has provided descriptive data to the published literature of sweat losses, and net body mass changes during training and competition. Some of these data were reviewed by for a Fédération Internationale de Football Association (FIFA) Medical Assessment and Research Centre meeting and it demonstrates clearly the substantial variability in sweating response and drinking behaviours even when players are doing the same training at the same time. This has also been shown to be the case in match play. Therefore, while some individuals may readily lose 2% or more of their body mass when sweating, other individuals may never or rarely reach this extent of body mass loss.

Hydration, Fluid Intake and Performance

Acute mild and moderate hypohydration can be relatively common in individuals exercising or who are exposed to warm environments due to the loss of sweat. It may also occur in situations of restricted fluid intake or due to consumption of diuretics. The effect of hypohydration on different types of exercise performance has been investigated including physical performance of strength, power and high-intensity endurance, endurance performance and skill accomplishment, cognitive performance, mood and mental readiness. In some of these areas, however, there are a relatively small number of scientific investigations which impacts on the strength of the conclusions that can be drawn. Nevertheless, the available evidence suggests that:

- Reductions in body mass in the order of 3–4% appear to consistently attenuate strength (by ~2%), power (by ~3%) and high-intensity endurance (by ~10%) suggesting that alterations in total body water do affect some aspect of muscle force generation.
- Reductions in body mass in the order of 2–3% appear to have no significant effect on sprint running performance, that is, when body mass is 'carried'.
- Reductions in body mass in the order of 2–7% significantly reduce endurance exercise performance, particularly in environments that are warmer than 30 °C.

- Reductions in body mass in the order of 1–2% appear to have no influence on endurance exercise performance when the exercise duration is less than 90 minutes and environment is temperate (20–21 °C).

In 2003, the International Olympic Committee held its second Consensus Conference on Nutrition for Sport. The conference considered the impact of hydration status on sport and exercise and concluded the following with regards to hydration in its consensus statement:

- Sodium should be included in fluids consumed during exercise if the exercise lasts more than 2 hours. It should also be included in fluids consumed by individuals in any event who lose more than 3–4 g of sodium in their sweat.
- Normally, before commencing exercise, euhydration should be ensured. Urine osmolality, specific gravity and colour are markers that can be used as a guide.
- After exercise that has resulted in body mass loss due to sweat loss, water and sodium should be consumed in a quantity greater than the losses to optimise recovery of water and electrolyte balance.

In addition to the hydration benefits imparted by drinking during exercise, ingestion of cold drinks has been shown to influence body temperature when exercising in moderate or warm environments and to improve exercise capacity in hot conditions.

Water, Sports Drinks and Other Drinks

Sports drinks mean different things to different people. In its simplest sense, a sports drink is a drink consumed in association with sport or exercise – either in preparation for exercise, during exercise itself or as a recovery drink after exercise. By definition, a drink is a liquid substance and as such, water is a main ingredient. However, a sports drink can contain a variety of nutrients and other substances. Therefore consumption of a sports drink will provide a large amount of water in addition to other components which could otherwise be obtained from food.

The formulation of sports drinks is related to that of oral rehydration solutions designed for the treatment of diarrhoea, in that water, carbohydrate and sodium are the key ingredients. The majority of mainstream sports drinks have a carbohydrate content close to 6% weight/volume and contain small amounts of electrolytes, the main one being sodium.

Table: The composition of selected UK based sports drinks and other beverages. Carbohydrate content is taken from drink labels. Other data from samples analysed in the laboratory.

	Carbohydrate (%)	Sodium (mmol/l)	Potassium (mmol/l)	Osmolality (mosmol/kg)
Gatorade	6	20	3	280
Isostar	7	30		289

Lucozade Sport	6.4	22	3	285
Powerade	6	23	2	280
Orange juice	10	4	45	660
Apple juice	13	1	26	
Tomato juice	3	10	7	
Cola	11	3	1	700
Oral rehydration solution	2	45	20	250
Bottled water	0	0	0	9
Milk	5	26	37	288

The main aims of sports drink consumption do vary according to the exercise situation, but, from a hydration point of view, are likely to be one or more of the following: to speed rehydration, to stimulate rapid fluid absorption, to reduce the physiological stress of exercise and to promote recovery after exercise.

Hydration during Exercise

In any exercise task lasting longer than about 30–40 minutes, carbohydrate depletion, elevation of body temperature and reductions in the circulating fluid volume may be important factors in causing fatigue. All of these can be manipulated by the ingestion of fluids, but the most effective drink composition and the optimum amount of fluid will depend on individual circumstances. Water is not the optimum fluid for ingestion during endurance exercise, and there is compelling evidence that drinks containing added substrate and electrolytes are more effective in improving performance. Increasing the carbohydrate content of a drink will increase the amount of fuel available, but will tend to decrease the rate at which water can be made available. Where provision of water is the priority, the carbohydrate content of a drink and its total osmolality should be low, thus restricting the rate at which substrate is provided. The composition of a drink will thus be influenced by the relative importance of the need to supply fuel and water, which in turn depends on the intensity and duration of the exercise task, on the ambient temperature and humidity and on the physiological and biochemical characteristics of the individual athlete. Carbohydrate depletion will result in fatigue and an inability to sustain exercise intensity, but is not normally a life-threatening condition. Disturbances in fluid balance and temperature regulation can have potentially serious consequences, and it may be therefore that the emphasis for many participants in endurance events should be on proper maintenance of fluid and electrolyte balance.

Carbohydrate

The optimum type and concentration of sugars in a drink will depend on individual circumstances. High carbohydrate concentrations will delay gastric emptying, thus reducing the amount of fluid that is available for absorption: very high concentrations will also result in secretion of water into the intestine and thus temporarily increase the likelihood of dehydration. Perhaps because of this effect, high sugar concentrations (>10%) may result in an increased risk of gastrointestinal disturbances. Where there is a need to supply an energy source during exercise, however, increasing the sugar content of drinks will increase the delivery of carbohydrate to the site of absorption in the small intestine.

Electrolytes

The available evidence indicates that the only electrolyte that may need to be added to a drink consumed during exercise is sodium, which is usually added as sodium chloride, but which may also be added as other salts e.g. sodium citrate. Sodium will stimulate sugar and water uptake in the small intestine and will help to maintain extracellular fluid volume as well as maintain the drive to drink by keeping plasma osmolality high. As is clear from table, most soft drinks of the cola or lemonade variety contain virtually no sodium (1–2 mmol/l), and water is also essentially sodium free; sports drinks commonly contain ~20–25 mmol/l sodium, and oral rehydration solutions intended for use in the treatment of diarrhoea-induced dehydration have higher sodium concentrations, in the range 30–90 mmol/l. A high sodium content may be important in stimulating jejunal absorption of glucose and water, but it may make drinks unpalatable.

Some degree of hyperthermia and hypernatraemia are relatively common in endurance events held in the heat. It has, however, become clear that a small number of individuals at the end of very prolonged events may be suffering from hyponatraemia: this may be associated with either hyperhydration or hypohydration. The total number of reported cases is small, and the great majority of these have been associated with ultramarathon or prolonged triathlon events. Many of the drinks consumed in endurance events, whether plain water, soft drinks or sports beverages, have relatively little or no electrolyte content. Most carbohydrate–electrolyte drinks intended for consumption during exercise have a low electrolyte content, with sodium concentrations typically in the range of 20–25 mmol/l. This is adequate in most situations, but may not be so when sweat losses and fluid intakes are high. Some supplementation with sodium chloride in amounts beyond those normally found in sports drinks may be required in extremely prolonged events where large sweat losses can be expected and where it is possible to consume large volumes of fluid. However, electrolyte replacement during exercise is not a priority for the majority of participants in most sporting events.

Cardiovascular, Metabolic and Performance Effects

Many of the published studies investigating the effects of fluid ingestion on exercise performance have failed to include appropriate controlled trials that allow the separate effects of water replacement and substrate provision to be assessed. Generally, the studies in the literature have reported either no effect of fluid ingestion on exercise performance or a beneficial effect. There seems to be a lessened hyperthermia and cardiovascular drift during prolonged moderate intensity exercise which is attributed to fluid replacement during the exercise. A better maintenance of blood glucose, which can be used by the exercising muscles with a consequent reduction in the need for mobilisation of the limited liver glycogen reserves, appears to be the major benefit of carbohydrate consumption during exercise. The studies that have reported adverse effects of fluid ingestion on exercise performance have generally been studies in which the fluid ingestion has resulted in gastrointestinal disturbances.

Drinking plain water can improve performance in endurance exercise, but there are further performance improvements when carbohydrate and electrolytes are added. The study of attempted to distinguish between the effects of carbohydrate provision from the water replacement properties of a drink. Eight men undertook the same cycle ergometer exercise on four separate occasions. After 50 minutes exercise at 80% of $VO2_{max}$, a performance test at a higher exercise intensity (completion of set amount of work as quickly as possible) was completed; this test lasted approximately 10 minutes. On each of the four trials, a different beverage consumption protocol was followed during the 50-minute exercise; nothing was consumed during the performance tests. The beverages were electrolyte-containing water in a large (1330 ml) and small (200 ml) volume and carbohydrate–electrolyte solutions (79 g) in the same large and small volumes; the electrolyte content of each beverage was the same, 619 mg (27 mmol) of sodium and 141 mg (3.6 mmol) of potassium, respectively. The results indicated that performance improved by 6.5% after consuming the large volume of fluid in comparison with the smaller volume and improved by 6.3% after consuming the carbohydrate-containing rather than carbohydrate-free beverages; the fluid and carbohydrate each independently improved performance and the improvements were additive. The mechanism for the improvements in performance with the large fluid replacement vs. the small fluid replacement was attributed to a lower heart rate and oesophageal temperature when the large volume was consumed. The authors were unable to identify the mechanism by which carbohydrate ingestion improved performance.

Hydration after Exercise

Until the electrolytes (particularly sodium) lost in sweat are replaced after exercise, water balance will not be effectively restored and maintained. We do not lose plain water when we sweat and plain water alone will not allow us to recover effectively.

Practical Issues

The quantity of electrolytes lost in sweat is highly variable between individuals and although the optimum drink may be one that matches equal quantities with the electrolyte loss, this is virtually impossible in a practical situation. Sweat composition and loss varies considerably between individuals, and also with environment and clothing worn and may be further influenced by the state of acclimation. However, a moderate excess of salt intake would appear to be beneficial as far as hydration status is concerned, without any detrimental effects on health, provided that fluid intake is in excess of sweat loss and that renal function is not impaired. Concerns over the possible adverse effects of a high salt intake on health have led some athletes to restrict dietary salt intake. For athletes with large sweat losses, sodium loss will be correspondingly high: loss of 5 litres of sweat with a sodium content of 50 mmol/l requires ingestion of almost 15 g of sodium chloride to restore balance. This amount of sweat can easily be lost in 2–3 hours of hard exercise in hot, humid conditions. Although the diet will make a major contribution to replacement, normal daily salt intake from food is only about 6–8 g for the UK population, about half of whom rarely or never add salt to food at the table. There is clearly a high risk of salt deficit when losses are high.

A properly formulated sports drink has a valuable role to play in the diet of many athletes. This is particularly true in situations where solid food is not available or not desired by the athlete or where hydration is the main concern.

During exercise, there are few situations where sports drinks have had a negative impact on exercise performance and where this has occurred, it is generally because of gastrointestinal distress rather than via another physiological mechanism. Provided appropriate quantities are consumed, drinking plain water is generally better than drinking nothing at all, but drinking a properly formulated carbohydrate electrolyte sports drink may allow for an improved exercise performance with benefits being gained from both its carbohydrate content and the water and electrolyte content.

In order to achieve effective rehydration after exercise in the heat, or heat exposure or any type of exercise sufficient to cause sweat loss, the rehydration beverage should contain moderately high levels of sodium (e.g. 50 mmol/l). A source of substrate is not necessary for rehydration, although a small amount of carbohydrate (<2%) may improve the rate of intestinal uptake of sodium and water, and a larger quantity of carbohydrate should not negatively impact post-exercise rehydration provided an appropriate volume for rehydration can be consumed. The volume of beverage consumed should be greater than the net volume of sweat lost in order to make a provision for the ongoing obligatory urine losses. The palatability of the beverage is of importance as many individuals lose substantial amounts of sweat and so need to consume large amounts of fluid to replace them and this is more likely to be achieved if the taste is perceived as pleasant.

Ultimately, the choice of drink to be consumed will depend on the individual and their particular circumstances. Replacement of substrate in addition to water and electrolyte losses may be of importance in the post-exercise period in preparation for a further bout of exercise. In terms of sustaining life, substrate (muscle and liver glycogen) depletion is unlikely to have an adverse effect in an otherwise healthy individual, but water depletion, if not replaced, may have serious consequences. The current generation of commercially available sports drinks are generally a good compromised formulation to meet the needs of many athletes in many different situations.

SPORTS SUPPLEMENTS

Sports supplements (also called ergogenic aids) are products used to enhance athletic performance that may include vitamins, minerals, amino acids, herbs, or botanicals (plants) — or any concentration, extract, or combination of these. These products are generally available over the counter without a prescription.

Sports supplements are considered dietary supplements. Dietary supplements do not require U.S. Food and Drug Administration (FDA) approval before they come on the market. Supplement manufacturers do have to follow the FDA's current good manufacturing practices to ensure quality and safety of their product, though. And the FDA is responsible for taking action if a product is found to be unsafe after it has gone on the market.

Critics of the supplement industry point out cases where manufacturers haven't done a good job of following standards. They also mention instances where the FDA hasn't enforced regulations. Both of these can mean that supplements contain variable amounts of ingredients or even ingredients not listed on the label.

Some over-the-counter medicines and prescription medications, including anabolic steroids, are used to enhance performance but they are not considered supplements. Although medications are FDA approved, using medicines — even over-the-counter ones in ways other than their intended purpose puts the user at risk of serious side effects. For example, teen athletes who use medications like human growth hormone (hGH) that haven't been prescribed for them can have problems with growth, and may develop diabetes and heart problems.

Lots of sports organizations have developed policies on sports supplements. The National Football League (NFL), the National Collegiate Athletic Association (NCAA), and the International Olympic Committee (IOC) have banned the use of steroids, ephedra, and androstenedione by their athletes, and competitors who use them face fines, ineligibility, and suspension from their sports.

The National Federation of State High School Associations (NFHS) strongly recommends that student athletes consult with their doctor before taking any supplement.

Some Common Supplements affect the Body

Whether you hear about sports supplements from your teammates in the locker room or the sales clerk at your local vitamin store, chances are you're not getting the whole story about how supplements work, if they are really effective, and the risks you take by using them.

Androstenedione and DHEA

Androstenedione (also known as andro) and dehydroepiandrosterone (also known as

DHEA) are prohormones or "natural steroids" that can be broken down into testosterone. Andro used to be available over the counter, but now requires a prescription.

When researchers studied these prohormones in adult athletes, DHEA and andro did not increase muscle size, improve strength or enhance performance.

Andro and DHEA can cause hormone imbalances in people who use them. Both can have the same effects as taking anabolic steroids and may lead to dangerous side effects like testicular cancer, infertility, stroke, and an increased risk of heart disease. As with anabolic steroids, teens who use andro while they are still growing may not reach their full adult height. Natural steroid supplements can also cause breast development and shrinking of testicles in guys.

Creatine

Creatine is already manufactured by the body in the liver, kidneys, and pancreas. It also occurs naturally in foods such as meat and fish. Creatine supplements are available over the counter.

People who take creatine usually take it to improve strength, but the long-term and short-term effects of creatine use haven't been studied in teens and kids. Research in adults found that creatine is most effective for athletes doing intermittent high-intensity exercise with short recovery intervals, such as sprinting and power lifting. However, researchers found no effect on athletic performance in nearly a third of athletes studied. Creatine has not been found to increase endurance or improve aerobic performance.

The most common side effects of creatine supplements include weight gain, diarrhea, abdominal pain, and muscle cramps. People with kidney problems should not use creatine because it may affect kidney function. People younger than 18 years old do not use creatine. If you are considering using creatine, talk with your doctor about the risks and benefits, as well as appropriate dosing.

Fat Burners

Fat burners (sometimes known as thermogenics) were often made with an herb called ephedra, also known as ephedrine or ma huang, which acts as a stimulant and increases metabolism. Some athletes use fat burners to lose weight or to increase energy — but ephedra-based products can be one of the most dangerous supplements. Evidence has shown that it can cause heart problems, stroke, and occasionally even death.

Because athletes and others have died using this supplement, ephedra has been taken off the market. Since the ban, "ephedra-free" products have emerged, but they often contain ingredients with ephedra-like properties, including bitter orange or country mallow. Similar to ephedra, these supplements can cause high blood pressure, heart attack, stroke, and seizures.

Many of these products also contain caffeine, along with other caffeine sources (such as yerba mate and guarana). This combination may lead to restlessness, anxiety, racing heart, irregular heart beat, and increases the chance of having a life-threatening side effect.

Will Supplements Make me a Better Athlete?

Sports supplements haven't been tested on teens and kids. But studies on adults show that the claims of many supplements are weak at best. Most won't make you any stronger, and none will make you any faster or more skillful.

Many factors go into your abilities as an athlete — including your diet, how much sleep you get, genetics and heredity, and your training program. But the fact is that using sports supplements may put you at risk for serious health conditions.

So instead of turning to supplements to improve your performance, concentrate on nutrition and training, including strength and conditioning programs.

GLUTAMINE

Glutamine is a conditionally essential amino acid widely used in sports nutrition, especially because of its immunomodulatory role. glutamine plays several other biological functions, such as cell proliferation, energy production, glycogenesis, ammonia buffering, maintenance of the acid-base balance, among others. Thus, this amino acid began to be investigated in sports nutrition beyond its effect on the immune system, attributing to glutamine various properties, such as an anti-fatigue role.

Fatigue is defined as the inability to maintain power output and strength, impairing physical performance. The main causes of fatigue are: accumulation of protons in the muscle cell, depletion of energy sources (e.g., phosphocreatine and glycogen), accumulation of ammonia in the blood and tissues, oxidative stress, muscle damage and changes in neurotransmitter synthesis, such as the increase in serotonin and the decrease in dopamine.

In order to delay the onset of fatigue and to improve athletic performance, several nutritional strategies have been applied. Since the mid-1980s and 1990s, the role of amino acids in the development of fatigue has been discussed, and evidence demonstrated that plasma glutamine concentrations and the glutamine/glutamate plasma ratio are reduced in athletes under chronic fatigue and overtraining syndrome, raising a question about the possible ergogenic effects of glutamine supplementation.

Glutamine could delay fatigue by several mechanisms: (i) it is one of the most abundant glycogenic amino acids in humans and animals, having a significant influence on the anaplerosis of the Krebs cycle and gluconeogenesis, (ii) through the activation of glycogen synthase, glutamine is considered as a direct stimulator of glycogen synthesis, (iii) this amino acid is the main non-toxic ammonia carrier, avoiding the accumulation of this metabolite , (iv) glutamine is also linked to attenuation of muscle damage and is considered an indirect antioxidant via stimulation of glutathione synthesis, among others.

Despite the potential of glutamine in attenuating some causes of fatigue, the effects of this amino acid supplementation on fatigue markers and physical performance have not been yet completely elucidated. Thus, the present article aims to review the main anti-fatigue properties of glutamine and the effects of this amino acid supplementation in this regard.

Glutamine and Physical Exercise

Glutamine is a five-carbon neutral amino acid, containing the molecular weight of 146.15 g/mol, and considered as the most abundant free amino acid in the human body. In adult humans following overnight fast, the normal blood levels of glutamine are 550–750 _mol/L , contributing for more than 20% of the blood amino acid pool. In the skeletal muscle, glutamine comprises 50–60% of the total free amino acid pool, being considered as the most synthesized amino acid in the human muscle, especially in slow-twitch muscles, which contain glutamine concentrations 3-fold higher than fast-twitch muscles. Therefore, skeletal muscle releases glutamine into the circulation at high rates, approximately 50 mmol per hour in the fed state.

Organs can be classified as producers or consumers of glutamine – skeletal muscles, lungs, liver, brain and adipose tissue present high activity of glutamine synthetase (an enzyme that synthesizes glutamine from ammonia and glutamate in the presence of adenosine triphosphate-ATP) and are considered as glutamine producers. On the other hand, leucocytes, enterocytes, colonocytes, thymocytes, fibroblasts, endothelial cells, and kidney tubular cells present high activity of glutaminase (an enzyme that hydrolyzes glutamine, converting it into glutamate and ammonia) and are classified as consumers of glutamine.

Organs can be classified as producers or consumers of glutamine – skeletal muscles, lungs, liver, brain and adipose tissue present high activity of glutamine synthetase (an enzyme that synthesizes glutamine from ammonia and glutamate in the presence of adenosine triphosphate-ATP) and are considered as glutamine producers. On the other hand, leucocytes, enterocytes, colonocytes, thymocytes, fibroblasts, endothelial cells, and kidney tubular cells present high activity of glutaminase (an enzyme that hydrolyzes glutamine, converting it into glutamate and ammonia) and are classified as consumers of glutamine.

Since the mid-1970s and 1980s, glutamine metabolism has been investigated during and after physical exercise , and it was observed that blood glutamine responds differently according to the duration of the exercise. Short-term exercise increases muscle release of glutamine and its blood concentrations , whereas, in long-term and exhaustive exercises, such as marathon race, muscle synthesis of glutamine is insufficient to meet the body need for this amino acid, decreasing blood glutamine. This decrease is transient and seems to last for 6–9 hours after a marathon , and is accompanied by a 30–40% fall in muscle glutamine or in its precursors, like glutamate. Nevertheless, it is worth mentioning that some studies demonstrated that even after exhaustive exercises (ultra-triathlon), blood glutamine did not change.

Decreased glutamine availability is linked with disorders in the immune system and an increase in the incidence of infections.

Regarding the glutamine supplementation, evidence indicates that plasma glutamine, in response to glutamine supplementation, increases markedly within 30 min after supplementation, returning to basal levels about 2 hours after glutamine administration. Moreover, doses of 20–30 g of glutamine have been reported to be tolerated (no side effects), offering no harm to humans.

Initially, glutamine was supplemented mainly because of its immunomodulatory potential. However, since this amino acid plays a wide variety of biological activities, glutamine began to be investigated in sports nutrition beyond its effect on the immune system, attributing to this amino acid several properties, such as an anti-fatigue role.

Glutamine and its Anti-Fatigue Properties

Fatigue is a multiple-cause phenomenon defined as the inability to maintain power output and strength, resulting in physical and mental performance impairment. Conceptually, fatigue may be classified as peripheral, also called muscle fatigue, when the biochemical changes occur within the skeletal muscle cell, or central, comprising disturbances in the central nervous system (CNS) that limit performance.

The main causes of fatigue are: (i) accumulation of protons in the muscle cell, reducing the pH and affecting the activity of enzymes, such as phosphofructokinase, (ii) depletion of energy sources (e.g., phosphocreatine and glycogen) for the continuity of the exercise, (iii) accumulation of ammonia (toxic metabolite) in the blood and tissues, (iv) oxidative stress, (v) muscle damage and (vi) changes in neurotransmitter synthesis, such as the increase in serotonin and the decrease in dopamine , which may cause a state of tiredness, sleep, and lethargy during prolonged exercises.

The underlying mechanisms behind the increase in brain serotonin are the plasma increase in its precursor, free (not albumin-bound) tryptophan, and the plasma decrease in the large neutral amino acids, such as branched-chain amino acids (BCAA), which compete with tryptophan to enter the brain. In addition, during long-term exercise, the augment in free fatty acid (FFA) concentrations can displace tryptophan from albumin, increasing free tryptophan and facilitating its brain influx and, consequently, serotonin synthesis.

Regardless of the origin (peripheral or central), fatigue is a complex and multifaceted phenomenon, since several factors may limit performance, but the improvement of single markers might not necessarily delay fatigue. Furthermore, it is worth highlighting that some causes of fatigue are not completely elucidated in the literature, such as the relationship between increased serotonin synthesis and performance decrease.

In order to delay the onset of fatigue and to improve athletic performance, several nutritional strategies are applied. Since the mid-1980s and 1990s, the role of amino acids in the development of fatigue has been discussed, and evidence demonstrated that blood glutamine and the glutamine/glutamate blood ratio were reduced after strenuous exercises, although some studies did not corroborate these findings.

Jin et al. observed a drastic decrease in plasma, muscle, and liver glutamine concentrations in an animal model of complex fatigue (forced swimming). Similarly, Kingsbury et al. verified that elite athletes under chronic fatigue (for several weeks) presented critical concentrations of blood glutamine (<450 μmol/L) and higher prevalence of infections compared to athletes without fatigue. An increase in protein intake (through lean meat, fish, cheese, milk powder and soya, that is, glutamine-rich foods) to these fatigued athletes enhanced blood glutamine levels and improved physical performance, raising the question about the possible anti-fatigue effects of glutamine supplementation.

Glutamine is one of the most abundant glycogenic amino acids in humans and animals, having a significant influence on the anaplerosis of the Krebs cycle and gluconeogenesis, being the most important energy substrate for renal gluconeogenesis. Additionally, glutamine is a direct stimulator of glycogen synthesis via the activation of glycogen synthetase, possibly through a mechanism of cell-swelling and to the diversion of glutamine carbon to glycogen, increasing hepatic and muscle glycogen stores.

Glutamine is also associated with the prevention of ammonia accumulation. Ammonia production during exercise occurs via amino acid oxidation and in energy metabolism (adenosine monophosphate-AMP deamination), indicating the reduction of ATP concentration and glycogen content ; thus, glutamine supplementation could minimize ammonia production due to its effects on energy metabolism. Ammonia accumulation is an important cause of fatigue since this metabolite is toxic and affects the activity of some flux-generating enzymes, the cell permeability to ions and the ratio of NAD+/NADH. However, as a consequence of the increase in ammonia production during exercise, glutamine synthesis is augmented, as a mechanism of ammonia buffering.

Glutamine may also attenuate ammonia accumulation because this amino acid is the main transporter of nitrogen (ammonia) in the body, preventing the muscle accumulation of this metabolite, and favoring ammonia hepatic metabolism, as well as its renal excretion.

Muscle damage and oxidative stress are other causes of fatigue that could be minimized by glutamine. Studies in our laboratory showed that glutamine supplementation (for 21 days) reduced the plasma concentrations of creatine kinase (CK) and lactate dehydrogenase (LDH)—markers of muscle damage—in rats submitted to strenuous resistance training. Several mechanisms might explain this protective effect of glutamine; this amino acid is absorbed through a sodium-dependent transport, increasing the intracellular concentration of sodium ions and promoting water retention, which increases cell hydration and its resistance to lesions. Glutamine also presents an important immunomodulatory role, increasing the synthesis of anti-inflammatory and cytoprotective factors, such as interleukin 10 (IL-10) and heat-shock protein (HSP).

Moreover, evidence indicates that glutamine is an important donator of glutamate for glutathione synthesis—the most important non-enzymatic antioxidant in the cell—which may indicate an indirect antioxidant effect of glutamine. Although elevated oxidative stress might contribute to fatigue, it is unclear in the literature whether the increase in glutathione concentrations through glutamine supplementation could attenuate fatigue and improve physical performance.

When glutamine is administered with alanine, as dipeptide (L-alanyl-L-glutamine), the fluid and electrolyte absorption seem to be even higher than supplementation with glutamine alone since dipeptide presents great stability in solution and low pH. Considering the potential properties presented, glutamine seems to be an interesting supplement for fatigue attenuation, especially for athletes who practice endurance sports (exhaustive and prolonged exercise). In figure, the main properties of glutamine in delaying fatigue are presented.

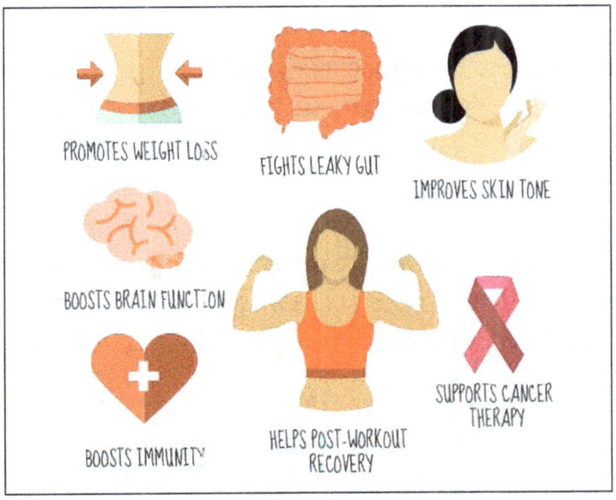
PROMOTES WEIGHT LOSS
FIGHTS LEAKY GUT
IMPROVES SKIN TONE
BOOSTS BRAIN FUNCTION
SUPPORTS CANCER THERAPY
BOOSTS IMMUNITY
HELPS POST-WORKOUT RECOVERY

Effects of Glutamine Supplementation on Exercise-Induced Fatigue Glutamine: The effects of glutamine infusion after an exhaustive exercise (cycling at 70–140% of the $VO2_{max}$ for 90 min) were first tested in 1995. Three groups of individuals were submitted to exercise and infusion (30 min after completing the exercise) of (i) glutamine, (ii) alanine and glycine or (iii) saline. Muscle glutamine concentrations were increased during glutamine infusion, reduced during alanine and glycine infusion and remained constant during saline infusion. Two hours after exercise, the muscle glycogen content was higher in the subjects treated with glutamine compared to other groups. It suggested that glutamine has effects on glycogen synthesis beyond its gluconeogenic role, since alanine and glycine, despite providing glucose through gluconeogenesis, did not affect muscle glycogen.

Similarly, Bowtell et al. investigated the effects of glutamine supplementation on whole body carbohydrate storage and muscle glycogen resynthesis in subjects after completing a glycogen-depleting exercise protocol. Individuals cycled on the ergometer at 70% of the $VO2_{max}$ for 30 min; thereafter, the workload was doubled and they completed 6 times of 1 min bursts of activity separated by 2 min of rest. Finally, they cycled for 45 min at 70% of the $VO2_{max}$. After exercise, individuals received one of the three drinks: (i) 18.5% glucose polymer solution, (ii) 18.5% glucose polymer solution containing 8 g of glutamine or (iii) a placebo containing 8 g of glutamine. Plasma glucose and insulin were higher when consuming drinks with glucose, and there was a tendency for plasma insulin to be higher after ingesting glucose and glutamine rather than only glucose. Supplementation with glutamine-containing drinks increased plasma glutamine. In the second hour of recovery, glucose and glutamine solution increased whole body non-oxidative glucose disposal by 25%, whereas oral glutamine alone promoted the storage of muscle glycogen to an extent similar to glucose. This result is surprising since it would be expected that the provision of 61 g of glucose polymer (amount of glucose provided in the glucose polymer solution), as opposed to 8 g of glutamine (amount of glutamine provided in the placebo solution), would result in a higher muscle glycogen synthesis; thus, it suggests a great impact of glutamine on muscle glycogen synthesis. However, there is limited evidence concerning this effect on glycogen synthesis in the athlete population.

The same research group, in 2001, observed a significant increase in the muscle concentrations of Krebs cycle intermediates, such as citrate, malate, fumarate and succinate, at the beginning of the exercise (bicycle exercise at 70% of the $VO2_{max}$) after acute glutamine supplementation, when in comparison with ornithine α-ketoglutarate or placebo administration. Nonetheless, glutamine supplementation did not affect the extent of phosphocreatine depletion, lactate accumulation or endurance time, suggesting that the muscle concentration of Krebs cycle intermediates was not limiting for energy production and physical performance.

Contrary to the abovementioned studies, van Hall et al. verified that the supplementation with free glutamine or a carbohydrate mixture containing glutamine did not affect muscle glycogen resynthesis after exercise. Individuals were submitted to an intense cycle ergometer exercise in order to deplete glycogen. Thereafter, subjects ingested four different drinks in three 500 mL boluses, immediately after exercise, 1 h after exercise and 2 h after exercise. The drinks were: 1—control: 0.8 g/kg of glucose, 2—glutamine: 0.8 g/kg of glucose plus 0.3 g/kg of glutamine, 3—a wheat hydrolysate containing 0.8 g/kg of glucose and 26% of glutamine, and 4—a whey hydrolysate containing 0.8 g/kg of glucose and 6.6% of glutamine. Plasma glutamine was reduced with control drink intake, remained unchanged with hydrolysates (wheat and whey) consumption and was 2-fold increased after glutamine supplementation. Despite increasing plasma glutamine, this amino acid administration did not improve glycogen synthesis rate. The different supplementation protocols and administered doses might explain the differences in the results of these studies.

Besides depleted glycogen stores, other markers of fatigue, such as blood ammonia and muscle damage parameters, were investigated after glutamine supplementation. Carvalho-Peixoto et al. supplemented glutamine and/or carbohydrate for high-trained runners before running for 120 min (~34 km), and observed that, contrary to placebo, there was no increase in blood ammonia in supplemented individuals in the first 30 min of exercise. Additionally, in the last 90 min of running, subjects under all supplementations had lower blood ammonia levels compared to placebo. There was no difference between supplementations, suggesting that glutamine and carbohydrate may attenuate ammonia increase during exercise, but without synergy between them.

Likewise, the effects of glutamine or alanine supplementation, either for short-term (1 day) or long-term (5 days), were investigated on blood ammonia of professional football players after two different exercise protocols—intermittent (a football match) or with continuous intensity (running for 60 min at 80% of the maximum heart rate-HRmax). Both exercises increased blood ammonia, whereas long-term glutamine supplementation protected against hyperammonemia only after the intermittent exercise, suggesting that the effect of glutamine administration on blood ammonia depends on the duration of the supplementation and on the type of physical exercise.

Different from these studies, Koo et al. compared the supplementation with glutamine, BCAA or placebo to elite rowing athletes that were engaged in a session of rowing (2000 m) at the maximal intensity, and observed that none of the interventions affected plasma ammonia, lactate and the cytokines IL-6 and IL-8; nevertheless, glutamine supplementation reduced the plasma levels of CK 30 min after exercise compared to the values measured immediately after training, suggesting a possible effect of glutamine in attenuating muscle damage.

Concerning the physical performance, Favano et al. supplemented glutamine peptide and carbohydrate or only carbohydrate to soccer players that were submitted to an intermittent exercise on the treadmill, and observed an increase in the time and distance (21% and 22%, respectively) and reduced rate of perceived exertion (RPE) after supplementing with glutamine and carbohydrate compared to the administration of only carbohydrate. Similarly, the supplementation with glutamine and carbohydrate to subjects that performed a running-based anaerobic sprint test (6 × 35 m discontinuous sprints) increased the maximal and minimal power compared to placebo (water + sweetener). Nava et al. also observed that glutamine supplementation reduced subjective fatigue, ratings of perceived exertion and gastrointestinal damage (measured by intestinal fatty acid binding proteins), besides increasing HSP70 and inhibitor of kappa B (IκBα) in peripheral blood mononuclear cells (PBMCs), in individuals submitted to a simulated wildland firefighting session in hot conditions.

In contrast to these studies, Krieger et al. verified that chronic glutamine supplementation did not improve performance during interval training. These data suggest that the combination of glutamine and carbohydrate is more efficient in preventing anaerobic power decrease and increasing performance than glutamine alone, emphasizing the synergy between glutamine and carbohydrate, although some studies did not corroborate this finding.

L-alanyl-L-glutamine

A high proportion of dietary glutamine is retained in intestinal cells, leaving only small concentrations of glutamine to enter into the bloodstream. In order to increase glutamine availability, the supplementation with peptides of glutamine, such as the dipeptide L-alanyl-L-glutamine, has been used, since di- and tripeptides are absorbed across the intestinal epithelium in their intact form by more efficient and faster mechanisms, such as the oligopeptide transporter PepT-1, than free amino acids. Thus, evidence showed that L-alanyl-L-glutamine supplementation was more effective in increasing plasma, muscle and liver glutamine concentrations compared to free glutamine administration. Furthermore, L-alanyl-L-glutamine presents higher stability in solution and low pH than glutamine and is a better option to be included in commercial products, such as sports drinks.

Rogero et al. supplemented glutamine (GLN) or L-alanyl-L-glutamine (DIP) for 21 days to rats submitted to swimming exercise for 6 weeks, followed by an exhaustion test. Animals were sacrificed immediately after the test (EXA) or after 3 h (REC). Muscle glutamine concentration was higher in DIP-EXA animals compared to CON-EXA and GLN-EXA groups, whereas DIP-REC group presented a higher plasma and liver content of glutamine than CON-REC group.muscle glutamine and protein levels were higher in GLN-REC and DIP-REC animals compared to CON-REC. Although supplementations, especially with L-alanyl-L-glutamine, increased glutamine concentrations, there were no differences between groups in the time to exhaustion, indicating that neither glutamine nor L-alanyl-L-glutamine supplementation improved physical performance.

Hoffman et al. administered L-alanyl-L-glutamine, in two doses (0.05 g/kg or 0.2 g/kg), or water to dehydrated male subjects (mild dehydration) submitted to an exercise session on the cycle ergometer at 75% of the $VO2_{max}$, and verified an increase in blood glutamine concentrations with the higher dose of dipeptide, as well as an increase in the time until exhaustion in both groups treated with L-alanyl-L-glutamine compared to water. There was no difference between trials in the parameters of muscle damage (blood CK), inflammation (blood IL-6), oxidative stress (blood malondialdehyde), among others. The authors attributed the performance improvement induced by L-alanyl-L-glutamine supplementation to the possible increase in fluid and electrolyte absorption promoted by this dipeptide; nonetheless, as seen previously, glutamine could delay fatigue through several other mechanisms, such as protecting against hyperammonemia.

The same research group investigated the effects of L-alanyl-L-glutamine, either in low (1 g/500 mL) or high dose (2 g/500 mL), on physical performance during a basketball game (jump power, reaction time, shooting accuracy and fatigue), and observed an improvement in basketball shooting performance and visual reaction time with low dose of L-alanyl-L-glutamine compared to water ingestion (placebo). Similarly, McCormack et al. submitted endurance-trained men to a one-hour treadmill run at 75% of the $VO2_{peak}$ followed by a run to exhaustion at 90% of the $VO2_{peak}$, after supplementing them with (i) L-alanyl-L-glutamine and a sports drink, (ii) only the sports drink (placebo) or (iii) without any supplementation (no hydration trial). The authors observed that plasma glutamine was higher and time to exhaustion was longer when supplementing with dipeptide compared to the no hydration trial, but there was no difference between L-alanyl-L-glutamine supplementation and the sports drink only (placebo).

Our research group also investigated the effects of glutamine and alanine supplementation, as dipeptide (L-alanyl-L-glutamine) or in their free form, to rats submitted to a resistance training protocol, consisting of climbing a vertical ladder with progressive loads. We observed that these interventions reduced parameters of muscle damage (plasma CK and LDH) and inflammation (plasma IL-1β and tumor necrosis factor alpha—TNF-α), and increased anti-inflammatory and cytoprotective markers (plasma IL-6, IL-10 and muscle HSP70). Additionally, these supplementations reduced the oxidized glutathione (GSSG)/reduced glutathione (GSH) ratio in erythrocytes and muscle thiobarbituric acid reactive substances (TBARS), evidencing an antioxidant role. Despite improving several parameters, glutamine and alanine administration did not improve performance evaluated by a maximum carrying capacity test.

In fact, recently, we observed that these amino acids supplementation improved some fatigue markers, such as muscle ammonia and glycogen, while impaired others, since L-alanyl-L-glutamine administration increased the hypothalamic concentrations of serotonin and the plasma concentrations of its precursor (tryptophan), although without affecting physical performance. It is worth mentioning that serotonin is considered as a parameter of central fatigue, since it is linked to behavioral alterations, such as reduced appetite, sleepiness, and fatigue, reducing the mental and physical efficiency. Fatigue is a complex phenomenon and the improvement or impairment of single markers may not necessarily affect performance.

Glutamine Associated with Other Nutrients

Studies also have evaluated the effects of glutamine, associated with several other amino acids, on fatigue markers. Ohtani et al. observed that an amino acid mixture (glutamine: 0.65 g—the amino acid in the highest concentration in the mixture—leucine, isoleucine, valine, arginine, threonine, lysine, proline, methionine, histidine, phenylalanine and tryptophan), when supplemented for 90 days to elite rugby players, improved reported vigor and earlier recovery from fatigue. Moreover, amino acids administration increased parameters of oxygen-carrying capacity, such as hemoglobin, red blood cells count, hematocrit and serum iron. After one year without the supplementation, all parameters returned to basal values, indicating the need for daily supplementation to maintain the effects. Some limitations of this study should be highlighted. Firstly, since several amino acids were ingested, it is not possible to attribute the effects to any of them, and, secondly, some of the results (such as reported vigor) were obtained by questionnaires. Thus, several factors could have affected the accuracy of the results.

The same research group, in the same year, evaluated this amino acid mixture for middle- and long-distance runners. The athletes were engaged in sustained exercise (running) for 2–3 h/day, 5 days/week, for 6 months. During this period, subjects received three 1-month treatments, separated by one month of washout. The treatments consisted of three different doses of the amino acid mixture: 2.2 g/day, 4.4/day and 6.6 g/day. The main effects were observed with the higher dose (6.6 g/day), which increased the physical condition score and markers of oxygen-carrying capacity (hematocrit, hemoglobin, and red blood cells count), while decreased serum CK, a marker of muscle damage and inflammation.

This amino acid mixture was also investigated on the recovery from muscle fatigue following eccentric exercise. Individuals were submitted to a session of eccentric training and, thereafter, they were allowed to recover for 10 days while supplementing with amino acids mixture or placebo. Measures of muscle strength (maximum isometric strength, maximum concentric strength, and maximum eccentric strength) in both elbow flexor and extensor muscles showed an earlier recovery from muscle fatigue when supplementing with amino acids compared to placebo. Additionally, maximum isometric strength was higher in amino acid trials than in the placebo, and most of the individuals reported less delayed muscle soreness with amino acids supplementation, indicating an ergogenic effect of this intervention.

Likewise, Willems et al. tested the supplement 'CycloneTM', which contains whey protein (30 g), glutamine (5.1 g), creatine (5.1 g) and β-hydroxy-β-methylbutyrate (HMB) (1.5 g), for subjects submitted to 12 weeks of resistance training, and observed that this intervention improved some performance parameters, such as the number of repetitions for 80% pre-training 1-RM for lateral pull and bench press, but not others, like maximum voluntary isometric force (MVIF), time to fatigue at 70% of the MVIF, peak concentric strength and 1-RM of lateral pull. The authors concluded that this multi-ingredient supplement improves the ability to perform some resistance training-specific tasks.

Corroborating these data, an interesting study observed that the voluntary intake of a solution containing BCAA (15.2 mmol/L of leucine, 9.9 mmol/L of isoleucine, 11.1 mmol/L of valine), glutamine (16.6 mmol/L), and arginine (13.9 mmol/L), rather than water, was positively correlated with timing and volume of exercise in rats exercised on running wheels, indicating a preference for this amino acid solution as a consequence of the exercise practice. In addition, the intake of these amino acids increased the BCAA/tryptophan plasma ratio and decreased the brain release of serotonin, a central fatigue parameter.

In opposition to the studies above mentioned, Kersick et al. did not verified any effect of a supplementation containing whey protein (40 g), glutamine (5 g) and BCAA (3 g) on performance (training volume, muscular endurance, muscular strength and anaerobic capacity), blood parameters (albumin, globulin, glucose, electrolytes, hemoglobin, lipid profile, creatinine, urea, etc.) and body composition of individuals submitted to 10 weeks of resistance training. The controversy between these results and those previously mentioned might be due to the different amino acid composition in the supplements offered, resulting in distinct properties of each supplement.

Besides being administered with amino acids, glutamine is also a component of supplements containing several nutrients, such as caffeine and creatine. Gonzalez et al. evaluated the effects of a pre-workout supplement containing glutamine, arginine, leucine, isoleucine, valine, taurine, β-alanine, creatine, glucuronolactone and caffeine (the concentration of each nutrient was not specified), administered 10 min before a resistance training session (four sets of no more than 10 repetitions of barbell squat or bench press at 80% of the 1-repetition maximum–1-RM), to resistance trained men. The authors observed an increase in the number of repetitions, in the average peak and in the mean power performance for all sets when ingesting the pre-workout supplement compared to placebo, but there was no difference between treatments in the reported feelings of energy, focus or fatigue.

Differently, Naclerio et al. compared the administration of a multi-ingredient supplement (containing carbohydrate 53 g, protein 14.5 g, glutamine 5 g, and carnitine 1.5 g) to carbohydrate alone, administered before, during and immediately after a 90-min intermittent repeated sprint test, but did not observe changes in physical performance. Plasma CK concentrations were lower 24 h after exercise when supplementing with multi-ingredient supplement compared to carbohydrate, whereas plasma myoglobin levels were lower 1 h after exercise in carbohydrate trial than placebo. The authors concluded that these interventions do not present an anti-fatigue effect, but can partially attenuate muscle damage.

The same research group, in a similar protocol, verified that this multi-ingredient supplement attenuated fatigue perception without improving performance in soccer players. One hour after the intermittent test, plasma myoglobin levels were lower when administering the multi-ingredient supplement and carbohydrate compared to placebo, whereas carbohydrate supplementation elicited lower neutrophil and monocytes concentrations than multi-ingredient and placebo. There was no difference between trials in other parameters, such as CK, IL-6 and lymphocytes count.

Although some of these interventions have presented interesting results, as they contain several nutrients, it is not possible to attribute these effects to any of them, except for their synergetic impact. It is important to emphasize that even in the studies where glutamine was supplemented with several other nutrients, this amino acid was offered in high doses, being, in most of the cases, one of the most prevalent amino acids in the administered supplements.

Furthermore, it is worth highlighting that there are important differences between the studies evaluated, such as the supplementation protocol (dose, supplementation with free glutamine or associated with other nutrients, etc.), the exercise protocol (short-term exercise and aerobic, long-term exercise and endurance or intermittent), characteristics of the volunteers (gender, age, physical activity level, etc.), among others, which might partially explain the controversial results obtained.

CREATINE

Creatine is a natural substance that turns into creatine phosphate in the body. Creatine phosphate helps make a substance called adenosine triphosphate (ATP). ATP provides the energy for muscle contractions. The body produces some of the creatine it uses. It also comes from protein-rich foods such as meat or fish.

Creatine is the most popular of these substances, believed to enhance muscle mass and help athletes achieve bursts of strength. Part of the reason for creatine's popularity might be its accessibility. Creatine powder, tablets, energy bars, and drink mixes are available without a doctor's prescription at drug stores, supermarkets, nutrition stores, and over the Internet.

Although creatine is a natural substance, it hasn't been well-studied over the long term. Researchers still aren't sure what effects it might have on the body, although there is evidence that in the short term, creatinine is safe for high-intensity resistance training.

How is Creatine used?

Back in the 1970s, scientists discovered that taking creatine in supplement form might enhance physical performance. In the 1990s, athletes started to catch on, and creatine became a popular sports supplement. The supplement is particularly popular among high school, college, and professional athletes, especially football and hockey players, wrestlers, and gymnasts.

Creatine is thought to improve strength, increase lean muscle mass, and help the muscles recover more quickly during exercise. This muscular boost may help athletes achieve bursts of speed and energy, especially during short bouts of high-intensity activities such as weight lifting or sprinting. However, scientific research on creatine has been mixed. Although some studies have found that it does help improve performance during short periods of athletic activity, there is no evidence that creatine helps with endurance sports. Research also shows that not everyone's muscles respond to creatine; some people who use it see no benefit.

Despite the popularity of creatine among young people, there has been very little research conducted in children under age 18. Of those studies, a few have suggested a positive effect but the overall evidence is inconclusive. In one study, teenage swimmers performed better after taking creatine; in another study, it helped high school soccer players sprint, dribble, and jump more effectively.

Researchers are studying whether creatine might also be useful for treating certain health conditions caused by weakened muscles, including:

- Heart failure and heart attack.
- Huntington's disease.
- Neuromuscular disorders, including muscular dystrophy and amyotrophic lateral sclerosis (ALS or Lou Gehrig's disease).

Creatine is also being studied as a way to lower cholesterol in people with abnormally high levels. Although early research has been promising, it's too early to say for sure whether creatine is effective for any of these conditions.

The use of creatine as a dietary supplement has become increasingly popular over the past several decades. Despite the popularity of creatine, questions remain with regard to dosing, effects on sports performance, and safety.

Directions for Use

Creatine Dosing

The recommendations regarding dosing of creatine supplementation as an ergogenic aid are varied. While many studies have reported promising results with building lean muscle mass or improvements in "quick burst" athletic performance, there are no firm guidelines regarding a supplementation regimen. A recent meta-analysis of creatine doses ranging from 0.07 g per kg body weight per day to 5 g/d revealed favorable outcomes for creatine with resistance training for increasing lean muscle mass.When comparing studies, it does not appear that these outcomes were dose-dependent. Hall and Trojian advise 0.03 g per kg per day as a maintenance dose, for 4 to 6 weeks on average, based on multiple reviewed studies.However, maintenance use of creatine has ranged from 28 days to 10 weeks. Most commercially available creatine supplements are packaged to contain between 4 and 5 grams of creatine per dose. While some of these supplements recommend once-daily dosing, many appear intentionally vague regarding recommended frequency or duration of dosing. These products are not regulated by the US Food and Drug Administration, and thus, individual products often contain unreliable or variable quantities of the desired supplement and may contain unintended ingredients such as banned substances.

A loading dose of creatine is often used prior to implementation of a daily maintenance dose. Some studies have indicated that creatine stores can be increased without a loading dose, albeit over longer periods of time. A commonly accepted loading dose regimen is 20 to 25 grams per day, divided 4 times daily for 5 to 7 days, with variability between recommended loading doses. The International Society of Sports Nutrition supports a loading dose of approximately 0.3 g per kg per day for at least 3 days. However, there is no consistency in loading dose recommendations in strength, frequency, or duration.

Effects on Exercise and Performance

Harris et al were the first to document increased muscle creatine concentrations of 20% with creatine supplementation in the form of creatine monohydrate. Creatine supplementation increases lean body mass as well as strength, power, and efficacy in short-duration, high-intensity exercises. These ergogenic effects have been studied extensively in the weight room and laboratory, with limited studies in active game play scenarios. A meta-analysis from 2003 including 100 studies demonstrated significant improvements in laboratory-based exercise but did not show improvements in sports-specific activities after short-term creatine supplementation. Other studies have shown no improvement with sports-specific activities related to simulated soccer participation, simulated wrestling, tennis, or swimming.

One of the ergogenic effects of creatine supplementation is increased body mass. A meta-analysis showed that approximately 64% of studies measuring body mass and/or body composition noted a statistically significant increase in lean body mass due to creatine supplementation. The increases in body mass were thought to be the result of increased intracellular water related to fluid shifts due to the osmotic properties of creatine. Increased body mass has been noted in those using a creatine supplement without participation in an associated exercise program. However, taking creatine in conjunction with a resistance training program yielded greater increases in body mass.

Studies on creatine supplementation demonstrate increases in performance and strength in short-duration, maximal-intensity exercises, as measured by 1-repetition maximum, muscular power, number of repetitions, muscular endurance, speed, and total force. Strength gains after 28 days between groups taking creating alone, creatine plus resistance training, and placebo plus resistance training showed all groups significantly increased ($P < 0.01$) bench and leg press muscular strength, with the creatine plus resistance training group improving significantly more than the group taking creatine alone. In meta-analyses of creatine supplementation on upper and lower extremity performance, increased strength performance related to creatine supplementation was noted for both the upper and lower extremity. There was improved performance with creatine supplementation in conjunction with a resistance training program, especially evident in those with no previous training history (defined as exercising less than 3 h/wk). Changes in performance were independent of age, sex, supplement dosage, and supplement duration. The meta-analysis focusing on upper extremity response to supplementation displayed the most significant strength increases, mainly at the pectoralis muscles (major and minor), with performances in bench press increasing by approximately 5.3% with creatine supplementation. Other studies have demonstrated similar improvements in bench-press performance.

Most team sports require a combination of aerobic and anaerobic activities, which necessitates a combination of strength and endurance. Peripheral fatigue as a result of aerobic training may potentially decrease strength and performance. Creatine supplementation may prevent loss of strength as a result of aerobic activity when combined with anaerobic activities in recreational athletes.

Results have been inconsistent overall with regard to an individual athlete's response to creatine supplementation. This may in fact be due to preloading of creatine. Athletes with a higher baseline level of creatine before supplementation are less likely to derive benefit than an athlete with a low baseline level of creatine. This likely explains why some athletes appear to be "responders" to creatine supplementation while others are "nonresponders."

Currently, the scientific literature best supports creatine supplementation for increased performance in short-duration, maximal-intensity resistance training with a noted effect on lean body mass. Whether these effects of creatine supplementation lead to improved performance on the field of play remains unknown.

Safety Concerns

Short-term use of creatine is considered safe and without significant adverse effects, although caution should be advised as the number of long-term studies is limited. The International Society of Sports Nutrition notes that "there is no scientific evidence that the short- or long-term use of creatine monohydrate has any detrimental effects on otherwise healthy individuals." They go on to say that "supplementation in young athletes is acceptable and may provide a nutritional alternative to potentially dangerous anabolic drugs."

Many theories regarding adverse effects of creatine have been proposed, including potential for renal damage, hepatic injury, and difficulty maintaining hydration. There have been theoretical concerns regarding potential effects of creatine supplementation on renal function. Multiple studies have examined serum creatinine levels, while none has indicated any evidence of increased serum creatinine in young, healthy individuals. There have been isolated case reports of athletes sustaining hepatic injury with creatine use. However, each of these cases involved excessive or inappropriate creatine use or multiple ergogenic aids and supplements. These adverse reactions have not been identified in larger, healthy populations taking creatine in appropriate therapeutic doses.

Creatine is known to cause mild water retention and decreased urinary volume due to its osmotic effect. This may result in temporary weight gain, particularly during the loading phase. Because of the increased intracellular water volume, there is an increased risk of compartment syndrome, muscle cramps, dehydration, or heat illness. However, none of these potential adverse reactions have been supported. The safety of creatine supplementation is unknown in children and adolescents.

PROTEIN

Protein is the favorite nutrient of athletes because of its ability to stimulate muscle protein synthesis. While the exact amount of protein for muscle growth is not certain it is possible that amounts greater than the recommended dietary allowance of 0.8 g/kg are needed, although the jury is still out. Its suggest 1.2 to 1.7 g/kg as the amount of protein needed to improve aerobic capacity through mitochondria synthesis and build muscle mass and strength. The timing of protein intake appears to be the most important factor in achieving positive training adaptations. The period immediately after exercise is currently considered the ideal time. High-quality protein sources that contain all of the essential amino acids appear to be the most anabolic. Athletes who consume high-protein diets should also ingest adequate fluids to help prevent dehydration and consume adequate fruits and vegetables to offset any urinary calcium losses that may occur when protein intakes are high.

Protein has long been the favored macronutrient for athletes. The logic is simple: if you want big muscles and muscle is made of protein, then eating more protein equals more muscle. This simple rationale is more fiction than fact, but it is difficult to convince athletes that protein is not the most important nutrient for sports performance. Flip through the pages of any health and fitness magazine, and it is easy to see why athletes worship at the altar of protein-men with bulging muscles who look like cartoon heroes and women with perfectly toned bodies without a drop of cellulite smile from the magazine pages and claim that the latest protein powder, shake, or supplement is all it takes to achieve the perfect body. It addresses protein quantity, quality, and timing of intake, as well as the myths surrounding the dangers of excess protein, and inherent difficulty in assessing how much protein is needed to build muscle and fuel performance.

Protein Quantity

Skeletal muscle makes up 40% to 45% of body weight and is the largest storage site for amino acids. However, muscle is more than just protein; it also contains water, fat, glycogen, and some minerals. One pound of muscle contains 70 to 105 g of protein, and to build a pound of muscle, it is estimated that 10 to 14 g of additional protein is needed each day, although others dispute this claim. In addition to possible growth of muscle, protein is a highly versatile nutrient and is involved in other functions that are crucial to sports performance: cell regulation, muscle repair, immune function, neurological function, nutrient transport, and structural support. Protein needs are affected by many factors: age, sex, energy intake, carbohydrate intake, exercise type, duration, and intensity, as well as training phase (novice vs trained). Practitioners most often suggest protein in the range of 1.2 to 1.4 g/kg per day for endurance athletes and 1.2 to 1.7 g/kg per day for strength athletes. However, most athletes are very likely to be involved in both endurance and strength activities, so a general range of 1.2 to 1.7 g/kg per day is frequently the shorthand recommendation in practice.

Guidelines for protein quantity were derived from nitrogen balance studies. As Phillips and colleagues pointed out in a 2007 review of protein requirements in athletes, nitrogen balance may be adequate for establishing protein needs to prevent deficiency, but it is likely inadequate to quantify optimal intakes for muscle adaptations needed by endurance or strength-trained athletes. Amino acid oxidation, another technique used in research to determine protein needs during exercise, is also not the perfect measure.

Assessing protein needs for active people is not an easy task. In determining protein needs for sedentary, healthy individuals, the recommended dietary allowance of 0.8 g/kg of body weight relied on nitrogen balance studies. An often forgotten caveat to protein requirements is that 0.8 g/kg is needed when positive energy balance is maintained. Frequently, athletes are not in positive energy balance because of the high caloric requirements for sports training and competition, and for aesthetic sports such as diving and gymnastics, energy is restricted to achieve a thin build. Female athletes are not immune to the social pressures to be thin, and frequently, body image concerns override adequate fueling for sport. At a 2007 Protein Summit, the conference was introduced by reminding the audience that the recommended dietary allowance is not a "requirement of an individual or even a mean for individuals" but is a level of nutrient intake that should be adequate for most individuals. Athletes are not looking for "adequate" intake; they want optimal intake. Athletes frequently make the assumption that "there is a linear relationship between the amount of protein ingested and resulting desirable adaptation of muscle." The bottom line is that, at present, we cannot pinpoint the exact protein needs of athletes with any degree of certainty.

Protein Quality

"Whey" better protein, "liquid egg whites," "soy" good, and even plain old chocolate milk all claim to be the best protein source for athletes. In addition, there are the claims for individual amino acidsVglutamine, arginine, and branched-chain amino acids (BCAAs) are all marketed to athletes as giving them special ability to stimulate muscle protein synthesis, provide substrates for fuel, and promote faster recovery.

Milk Protein

The dairy industry has long promoted the health benefits of milk but focusing mostly on the micronutrients of calcium, vitamin D, and potassium. To stimulate muscle protein synthesis, weight training or resistance exercise provides a signal for growth, but without adequate nutrient substrate, maximal growth cannot be achieved. In the mid-1990s, researchers begin to look at the effects of various proteins on absorption and appearance in the blood. Boirie and colleagues studied milk proteins, whey, and casein, to assess how quickly amino acids appeared in the blood after acute feeding of labeled proteins. Whey protein makes up 20% of milk proteins, with casein providing about 80% of protein. Boirie et al showed that whey protein was highly soluble and was a "fast" protein, meaning that after whey protein feeding, the appearance of amino acids in the blood are fast, high, and transient. Casein, a "slow" protein, clots in the stomach, delaying gastric emptying, leading to a slower, lower, but more prolonged appearance in the blood after ingestion.

The dairy industry promoted the advantages of milk protein as unique in containing both fast and slow proteins, which theoretically could provide an advantage for muscle protein synthesis. The theory was simple-whey protein could stimulate protein synthesis but did not appear to affect protein breakdown, whereas the casein in milk could inhibit protein breakdown. It was sort of a "one-two punch" for muscle building simply by drinking a glass of milk.

Several researchers have since shown that milk proteins make for a good muscle building supplement. Wilkinson and colleagues compared milk protein with soy protein on muscle protein accretion. Young, healthy, resistance-trained men consumed isocaloric and isonitrogenous beverages of either soy protein or fluid skim milk after resistance-training leg exercises. The subjects completed 2 trials in random order, and blood flow, amino acid blood levels, and muscle biopsies were analyzed for markers of muscle protein synthesis. Researchers concluded that both the milk and soy proteins resulted in net protein muscle synthesis but that there was a greater rate of muscle mass accrual after milk protein ingestion. The authors believe that milk protein has a unique ability to sustain higher blood levels of amino acids than soy protein, and the prolonged elevation of amino acids in the blood results in a more favorable environment for muscle growth.

A recent abstract supports previous findings about milk protein when used as a recovery beverage in competitive soccer players. Thirteen college soccer players were given either chocolate milk or a carbohydrate energy drink (isocaloric) after intense training and soccer skill tests. The low-fat chocolate milk drinkers had lower levels of creatine kinase-a marker to measure muscle breakdown-than the carbohydrate beverage consumption. However, there was no difference in performance measures in the soccer players when the 2 different beverages were consumed.

Pros and Cons of Various Protein Supplements Commonly used by Athletes

Milk Protein

- Pros

  Contains both "fast" and "slow" proteins with 80% casein and 20% whey protein; Chronic consumption after weight training appears to support lean mass accrual more than other types of protein; Inexpensive; Taste is familiar to athletes; Milk contains carbohydrate and many other nutrients.

- Cons

  Whole milk contains saturated fat and cholesterol; All milk contains lactose so is not good for lactose-intolerant athletes; Requires refrigeration; Some athletes complain of "cotton mouth" after drinking milk.

Whey Protein

- Pros

  'Fast" protein, meaning, that it is rapidly digested, leading to increased amino acids in blood and stimulating protein synthesis; May improve immune function; May have antioxidant function; May decrease cardiovascular disease risk; May decrease risk of high blood pressure.

- Cons

  Whey protein and whey protein concentrate can contain lactose (whey protein isolate is lactose-free); Expensive; Powders have to be mixed with water.

Soy Protein

- Pros

  Protein quality comparable to animal protein; Considered a fast protein; Some forms of soy provide isoflavones; May reduce prostate cancer risk.

- Cons

  May not build muscle as rapidly compared with whey and casein; Taste may be unfamiliar to athletes; "Bad" press with soy protein (increases breast cancer risk, estrogen-like properties) may influence athletes to avoid soy protein.

Egg Protein

- Pros

  Considered the "perfect" food because of essential amino acid profile; Contains 13 other essential nutrients; Egg whites are fat-free, cholesterol-free.

- Cons

  Egg yolk is high in cholesterol, and half of the protein in egg is found in yolk; Raw eggs can be a source of Salmonella; Some athletes may be allergic to eggs.

Whey Protein

Whey protein is one of the most popular (and most advertised) protein supplements to athletes. Does whey protein have an advantage over milk protein's whey and casein? Tang and colleagues wanted to know if whey protein did indeed live up to its hype by studying the effect in the postexercise period in resistance-trained subjects. This is an important distinction because many studies with protein supplementation are conducted with untrained subjects-in studies that enrolled untrained subjects, the results of supplementation are almost universally positive, but can the same be said when individuals are already accustomed to weight training? In a double-blind, randomized, crossover trial involving leg extension to maximal resistance, young resistance-trained men were given 1 of 2 isocaloric beverages-carbohydrate-only or whey protein plus carbohydrate. Results, based on tracer injections, showed that whey protein plus carbohydrate induced greater muscle protein synthesis compared with the carbohydrate trial.

It is also important to note that the amount of protein needed to stimulate muscle growth is not large-more is not necessarily better when it comes to muscle growth-10 g of whey protein plus about 20 g of carbohydrate was sufficient to build muscle.

What is so special about whey protein compared with other protein supplements? Researchers believe that the key could be the amino acid leucine, one of the BCAAs. Whey protein has the highest amount of BCAAs of any protein. After exercise, leucine stimulates signaling pathways to stimulate muscle protein synthesis. Norton and Layman reported that leucine serves as a crucial regulator of protein synthesis and is donor of nitrogen to alanine and glutamine, 2 important amino acids in muscle protein synthesis. Researchers are excited about this "leucine trigger," as it may have important implications not only for muscle growth for healthy athletes but also for prevention and treatment of sarcopenia or age-related loss of muscle and function in older adults.

Egg Protein

Egg has often been called the "perfect protein" because of its amino acid profile and has been used as the standard for comparing other dietary proteins. Eggs are also rated high on digestibility, so combined with its amino acid content, it is an excellent source of protein for athletes. Eggs are a familiar food to athletes, but maybe, that familiarity makes them seem mundane, especially when other dietary supplements have more aggressive marketing campaigns. Eggs also have the bad reputation of being an unhealthy heart food based on cholesterol concentrations. One large egg has 75 cal, 6 g of protein, and 213 mg of cholesterol, but only 1.5 g of saturated fat; however, the egg white provides all of the amino acid benefits without the cholesterol. One large egg white has 16 cal with 3.5 g of protein and is fat-free. Research using eggs as the protein source for muscle growth is lacking, perhaps because of less available research funding from the egg producers when compared with the money from the dairy industry. However, egg protein is clearly a high-quality source of protein, but it takes 4 or 5 eggs to get the 10 g of essential amino acids that appear to be needed for stimulating protein sythesis.

Soy Protein

Soy protein is a high-quality protein that provides all of the essential amino acids needed for protein synthesis. Soy protein can be used by vegetarian athletes as a good alternative to meat and dairy foods to meet their protein needs. Soy protein powder is also available as a muscle-building supplement. Candow and colleagues studied soy protein (1.2 g/kg of body weight) on untrained young adults and compared it with whey protein (also at 1.2 g/kg) and found that both soy and whey protein increased lean mass compared with placebo. Other researchers have shown that whey protein is superior to soy protein for muscle anabolism, but the results should not be interpreted that soy protein has no effect on muscle growth. However, Candow et al used untrained subjects, and one would expect that muscle gains are greater in untrained subject versus trained subject whether ingesting soy or whey protein.

Protein Timing

One of the most important aspects of protein intake and muscle protein synthesis revolves around the timing of protein intake relative to exercise. Exercise, whether resistance or endurance activity, requires protein to aid in the adaptations that the athlete seeks. Weight lifters want an increase in size and strength of muscle fibers, and endurance athletes want more and bigger mitochondria to improve oxidative capacity. Resistance exercise leads to muscle trauma. Nosaka notes that muscle damage can be classified as 3 different types: muscle soreness, occurring 24 to 48 hours after exercise and often called delayed onset muscle soreness; acute damage from a minor to a major tear in muscle fibers; and muscle soreness or a cramp that happens during or immediately after exercise. The amount of muscle damage that athletes sustain in training may not be severe, but muscle damage does occur during and after exercise, so recovery is an important aspect of athletic training.

Most of the research on protein timing focuses on the postexercise period. Most researchers would agree that protein ingestion, either as food, supplements, or amino acids, in the period immediately after exercise (usually defined as within 1 hour) is an effective nutrition plan to minimize protein breakdown, stimulate muscle protein synthesis, and therefore aid in building muscle.

Humi and colleagues looked at timing of protein intake both before and after resistance training in young men. They measured muscle area using magnetic resonance imaging and performed muscle biopsies before and after 21 weeks of weight training and a control period. Using 15 g of whey protein given both before and after training, they found increased muscle area in all supplementation phases, but more of benefit (as measured by markers of protein breakdown) when protein was ingested after exercise. They concluded that protein intake timed around resistance exercise is more advantageous than protein intake at other times of the day.

However, Humi et al used untrained men in his study. Hoffman et al studied 10 weeks of protein supplementation on about 30 resistance-trained men. In this study, a higher dose of commercial protein supplement was used than in other studies (42 g of a blend of collagen, whey, and casein along with 2 g of carbohydrate) and was compared with a control group with no supplementation. Outcome measures included body composition analysis (dual-energy x-ray absorptiometry) and strength exercises performed to 1 repetition maximum. After 10 weeks, no differences between body composition or strength were seen between groups, suggesting that those individuals who are resistance trained will gain no further benefits from ingesting additional protein either before or after exercise.

Excess Protein and Health

One concern that always comes up when talking about excess protein are potential health risks. Will excess protein harm the kidneys or leech calcium from bones leading to an increase in fracture risk? While research on high protein consumption and specific athlete populations is limited, a few studies have shown that high-protein intakes do not have adverse effects on renal function as measured by glomerular filtration or creatinine clearance in healthy body builders. Both studies were conducted in Europe, and it would be helpful to have additional research in a US athlete population to assess the impact of a high-protein diet on renal function.

Bone volume is made up of about 50% protein and about one-third of its mass. Early studies showed that, for every gram of excess protein consumed, there is a 1-mg loss of urinary calcium. Heaney and Layman note that the frequently cited study was done using purified amino acid injections-not food sources of protein. With high-protein diets, up to 30% of energy as protein, there is a slight increase in urinary calcium excretion, but there is also an increase in intestinal calcium absorption. Protein consumption (in the range of 1.0Y1.5 g/kg) is associated with an increase in insulinlike growth factor 1, which is osteotrophic. One concern with high-protein intake on bone health is the effect on acid-base balance. A high protein, "Western"-type diet is acid forming and is associated with calcium loss in the urine. Calcium gets recruited from bone to buffer the acid and over time can contribute to bone loss. To negate this negative impact, adding fruits and vegetables to the diet can be an effective strategy.

Overlooked in the discussion of high intake of dietary protein are its effect on hydration and the potential to displace carbohydrate. At intakes greater than 2.5 g/kg, urea production from deamination can contribute to dehydration. Urea is osmotically active and draws water into the kidney tubules, increasing urine output and decreasing total body water. Carbohydrate, critical for aerobic and endurance exercise, is also important in strength training. Muscle glycogen reduction is seen after weight training, and in weight-lifting sessions that last an hour or longer, carbohydrate ingestion improves performance. All athletes should balance protein intake with sufficient carbohydrate intake and adequate fluids for peak performance, as well as long-term health.

SPORTS DRINK

Sports drinks are beverages that are specially formulated to help people rehydrate during or after exercise. They are usually rich in carbohydrates - the most efficient source of energy. As well as carbs, which are important in maintaining exercise and sport performance, sports drinks usually contain sweeteners and preservatives.

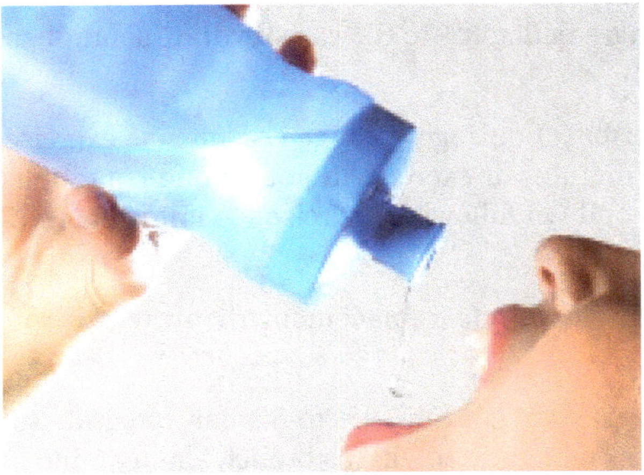

Sports drinks are often rich in carbohydrates.

Sports drinks also contain electrolytes (minerals such as chloride, calcium, magnesium, sodium and potassium), which, along with body fluid, diminish as you exercise and sweat.

Replacing the electrolytes lost during training promotes proper rehydration, which is important in delaying the onset of fatigue during exercise.

Keeping rehyrdated is particularly important for people with diabetes who have an increased risk of dehydration due to high levels of blood glucose.

Sports drinks have reached mainstream consumption, but their calories and nutrients are formulated for the sports market—not daily consumption, unless there is regular fluid and electrolyte loss. Sports drinks are designed to help delay the onset of fatigue during exercise and help rehydrate athletes after training or competition by replenishing carbohydrates, electrolytes, protein, and other nutrients. Most sports drinks provide a readily absorbable form of carbohydrates, important to exercising muscles, since carbohydrates are the primary fuel for exercise and are critical to performance.

Overconsumption of plain water can cause water intoxication or hyponatremia, an electrolyte disturbance in which the sodium concentration in blood plasma is too low. Severe or rapidly progressing hyponatremia can result in swelling of the brain and death. Fluids that supply 60 to 100 calories per 8 ounces help prevent this condition and provide needed carbohydrates, calories, electrolytes, and fluids for continuous performance, especially in extreme conditions over three hours.

Sports drinks come in a variety of colors with just as great a variety of ingredients. Some of the more popular types of sports drinks, typical ingredients, and optimal time of use are listed as follows:

- Carbohydrate-electrolyte replacement drink:
    - Typical ingredients: 4% to 8% carbohydrate solution, sodium chloride, and potassium.
    - Optimal use: (1) during prolonged or intense exercise lasting longer than 60 to 90 minutes or exercise in hot, humid conditions where sweat losses are high; and (2) following exercise for immediate fluid and carbohydrate replacement.
- Carbohydrate-electrolyte replacement drink with protein or other added nutrients:
    - Typical ingredients: Water, 4% to 8% carbohydrate solution, sodium chloride, potassium, and protein (as branch chain amino acids), as well as possibly herbs or caffeine, or both.
    - Optimal use: Research is not conclusive about the benefits of adding protein or caffeine to a sports drinks; however, if tolerated by an athlete, these ingredients could be used (1) during prolonged or intense exercise lasting longer than 60 to 90 minutes or exercise in hot, humid conditions where sweat losses are high; (2) following exercise for immediate fluid and carbohydrate replacement. To date there is no scientific support for a performance benefit or long-term safety data regarding the addition of protein or herbs to sports drinks. Caution should always be taken when consuming herbal ingredients, which can place athletes at risk for an adverse reaction or put them in violation of banned substance codes for their sport.
- Sports water:
    - Typical ingredients: Water, 2.5% to 3.8% carbohydrate solution (no carbohydrate if artificially sweetened), sodium chloride, B-vitamins, vitamins E and C.
    - Optimal use: (1) general everyday fluid replacement, (2) fluid replacement during shorter duration (<60 to 90 minutes), easy to moderate intensity exercise, especially if an athlete desires a change from drinking plain water. Although sports water may encourage fluid intake in athletes, there is no scientific support that vitamins will enhance exercise performance.

- Meal replacement drink:
  - Typical ingredients: Mixture of water, carbohydrates, protein, and sometimes fat; tend to be concentrated source of calories.
  - Optimal use: Ideal as a liquid preexercise or postexercise snack; may work well with an athlete too nervous to eat solid food before training or competition; however, caution should be taken when consumed before exercise that beverage is not consumed too close (<1 hour) to onset of exercise, which can lead to stomach distress in susceptible athletes.
- Energy drinks:
  - Typical ingredients: Water, carbohydrates, caffeine, sometimes herbs, protein (amino acids), electrolytes, vitamins, and minerals.
  - Optimal use: Not for use immediately before, during, or after exercise. The high carbohydrate content (sugar) in combination with carbonation prevents optimal hydration or rehydration. The high caffeine content could cause jitters and stomach distress if consumed too close to exercise. Herbal ingredients can place athletes at risk for an adverse reaction or put them in violation of banned substance codes for their sport. Scientific support for a performance benefit and long-term safety data regarding the addition of protein to a sports drink are lacking.
  - Overall, the perfect sports drink does not exist: The athlete must consider several factors when choosing a sports drink including the type of exercise to be performed (e.g., if glycogen depleting, carbohydrates should be a main ingredient in the sports drink); duration of exercise; intensity of exercise; tolerability; and of course, the preference of the athlete.

The Role of Sports Drinks and Hydration

During exercise the working muscles produce heat and this heat must be dissipated in order to keep the body temperature within safe limits.

Sweating, and its evaporation from the skin, is our most effective mechanism for regulating body temperature. If fluid lost as sweat is not replaced during exercise, the resulting dehydration quickly impairs performance. As little as a 2% of body weight lost as fluid (i.e. 1.5 litres for an average 75kg male) can result in a decrease in both mental performance (e.g. reduced concentration/decision making ability) and physical performance (fatigue/reduced muscular strength).

Replacing lost fluid is thus vitally important both for maintaining sporting performance and also for minimizing risks to health. Sports drinks have been specially designed to contain both carbohydrate and electrolytes which work to promote rapid absorption from the small intestine and increase retention of ingested fluid.

Ingredients in Sports Drinks

Sports drinks have three basic ingredients:

- Water,
- Sugar,
- Salt.

These three ingredients work to rehydrate, reenergise and replace lost electrolytes.

Hydration

The sugar and salt in sports drinks are at the right concentrations to maximise the speed with which water moves from your gut into your bloodstream. But plain water is absorbed almost as quickly and is perfectly adequate for moderate exercise or if you're exercising for less than about an hour.

But the sense of thirst is slow to react to dehydration, so if you're exercising hard in hot conditions it's a good idea to drink before you become thirsty. In fact you need to drink before, during and after exercise.

Energy

The sugars in sports drinks can also help replenish the fuel you use during exercise. The body stores fuel as carbohydrates in the muscles and the liver and releases sugar into the bloodstream for instant energy. But after prolonged exercise – about an hour of intense exercise, like a fast run or hard cycling – the carbohydrate stores are depleted and blood-sugar levels can drop. A steady source of sugar during strenuous exercise for an extended period can help fight off fatigue and enhance performance. With lower intensity exercise, such as jogging, it may take two hours or more before energy needs replacing.

Electrolytes

The salts in sports drinks help replenish the body's electrolytes lost in sweat. Sodium helps regulate the body's fluid balance and plays a role in muscle contraction, and potassium is also involved in muscle contraction. But for the average exerciser this is less important than the ads would have you believe: most of us already get too much salt in our regular diet so your usual food intake should be more than enough to replace any electrolyte losses. A 600mL bottle of some sports drinks gives you more than 10% of the maximum recommended daily intake of sodium.

However, for endurance athletes, sodium losses are a more serious issue: low sodium levels often coupled with excessive water consumption have caused more than a few deaths among athletes, hikers, military personnel and people undertaking strenuous activities over long periods of time in hot conditions

Kids and Sports Drinks

Sports drinks are sometimes promoted as better than water for young kids because the kids tend to drink more than if they were only offered water, preventing dehydration. But sports drinks are acidic and can erode dental enamel. And the salt in sports drinks is even more undesirable for children than it is for adults because their maximum recommended intake is less (depending on age).

TYPES OF SPORTS DRINKS

Isotonic Drinks

A drink is isotonic when it contains the same particulate concentration as blood. In order to determine this, we study the osmolarity of the drink, which must be between 270 and 330 mOsml / litre in order to be isotonic. So, a drink is hypotonic when less concentrated than blood and hypertonic when more concentrated.

Ingredients of Isotonic Drink

Water is the main ingredient of the drink. It ensures hydration during effort.

- Carbohydrates to ensure energy intake and enable continuous physical effort. The quantity of carbohydrates in a drink must be between 60 et 80 g / litre.
- Sodium to recover salts lost in sweat. In addition, sodium triggers a sensation of thirst and makes it easier to assimilate water and carbohydrates.
- Group B vitamins to facilitate the transformation of into energy and help combat fatigue.
- Potassium is useful in hot or warm weather.
- Magnesium to help reduce fatigue.
- Antioxidants to help the body defend itself against certain toxic waste produced by cell activity.
- There may be protein in the drink, but this is rare. It may be helpful over long periods of effort, i.e. more than 3 hours.

When should you have an Isotonic Drink?

Endurance sports, such as triathlon, involve a risk of dehydration through perspiration. Sweat is composed of water and minerals (mainly sodium, but also a little potassium).

During effort, the body may lose over one and a half litres in perspiration an hour, and sometimes up to 3 litres an hour. So, unless this loss is balanced by drinking, the body becomes dehydrated. Moreover, we know that muscles use energy during effort, so regular carbohydrate intake enables us to make up for losses and maintain effort.

Isotonic drinks are the best solution, since they provide water, sodium and carbohydrates. They are 'all-in-one' drinks.

After an hour of effort, you will thus need to drink isotonic drinks regularly. The required dose is 1 mouthful every 10-15 minutes from the start of your effort.

Health Benefits of Isotonic Drinks

Vigorous exercise helps promote heart health, weight loss and overall fitness, but it can also make you sweat one to three quarts of fluid during intense workouts. Although sweating is your body's way to help keep its core temperature cool, it can lead to the loss of important minerals, dehydration and heat stroke. Isotonic drinks replace those nutrients and fluids quickly, helping to prevent exercise-related injuries and illness.

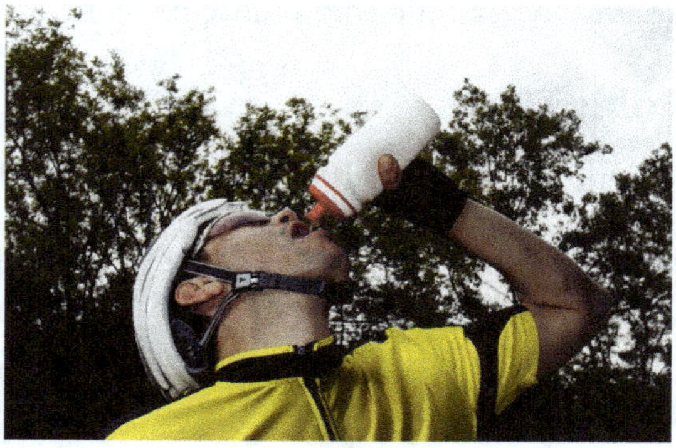

Identification

Sports drinks are classified three ways: isotonic, hypotonic and hypertonic, depending upon the amount of carbohydrates they contain. Isotonic fluids have six to eight percent carbohydrates, including glucose Isotonic drinks have an osmolality of 280 to 330 mOsm/kg, a measure of the number particles of carbohydrates, electrolytes, sweeteners and preservatives in a fluid. The osmolality rating of isotonic drinks best approximates that of your body's natural fluid balance, which is one reason why these drinks are so popular among runners and other endurance athletes.

Electrolytes

Electrolytes are essential minerals that help maintain the acid-base balance in your body's cells of sodium, potassium, calcium, magnesium, chloride, bicarbonate, phosphate and sulphate. Subjects given the isotonic drink retained more sodium, magnesium and calcium in their bodies enough to compensate for urinary and sweating losses.

Glucose

The carbohydrates glycogen, which is converted to glucose and stored in your liver/muscles, requires less oxygen to be burned for fuel than protein or fat. In a typical male athlete, for example, the liver stores 90 g of glycogen and the muscles store 400 g. During hard exercise, carbohydrate stores can be depleted at a rate of three to four grams per minute, which can almost exhaust your body's supplies in exercise sustained at two hours or more. It would ordinarily take 24 to 48 hours for your body to naturally replenish those supplies, but an isotonic drink can return the glycogen balance to your body much more quickly.

Hydration

It would seem logical to consume water during exercise when you're sweating, but water can cause bloating and it doesn't contain carbohydrate or electrolytes. The higher the carbohydrate level in a drink, the slower the rate of stomach emptying. Isotonic drinks empty from the stomach at a rate similar to water, reducing urine output and encouraging fluid retention to prevent dehydration.

Hypotonic Drinks

Hypotonic drinks have a lower concentration of carbohydrates (<5%) and salt than blood. This means they are absorbed into the bloodstream at a faster rate for quick hydration and electrolyte release. Hypotonics may contain carbohydrates too, helping to contribute towards your total energy intake. They are best for rapid hydration. When to use: Pre-hydration, on shorter workouts, on long rides, in hot weather; when you need a drink to rehydrate quickly & effectively.

Working Principle of Hypotonic Drink

When we drink a hypotonic drink the solution moves via osmosis across the gut walls and into the blood vessels. This means fast rehydration, as the drink is rapidly absorbed across the gut lining and quickly replaces fluids lost. There's a much lower risk of bloating, cramps and the dreaded GI distress that can come with other energy drinks too.

Hypotonic drinks will also give us a speedy top up of electrolytes – those vital salts and minerals lost in sweat – to help regulate muscle function and keep your fluid levels balanced.

Disadvantages of Hypotonic Drinks

Hypotonic drinks focus on rehydration and therefore do not provide maximum carbohydrates (energy). If you're out on a Sunday long run or have an epic day in the saddle planned, use these drinks in combination with your other nutrition, such as a Veloforte bar or an energy gel.

Hypertonic Drinks

Hypertonic sports drinks contain a higher concentration of salt and sugar than the human body and higher levels of carbohydrate than isotonic drinks. These are used to supplement daily carbohydrate intake normally after exercise, in order to top up muscle energy stores. Athletes who take part in ultra distance events, where sustained high levels of energy are required, use these drinks. Hypertonic drinks can be taken during exercise allowing the athlete to meet their energy requirements. They are normally used in conjunction with isotonic drinks to maintain fluids.

Working Principle of Hypertonic Drink

Hypertonic drinks provide the highest dose of carbohydrates (>8%) of all energy drinks. Despite a slower absorption rate than hypotonic or isotonic drinks, they're still a quick way to top up glycogen stores, as the body tends to absorb liquids more quickly than solid food.

Disadvantages of Hypertonic Drinks

Hypertonic drinks can cause dehydration as the body has to move water from the bloodstream into the intestine to dilute the fluids before it can absorb them. This can make you feel thirsty and sometimes nauseous. While some ultra athletes use hypertonic drinks alongside other hydrating drinks during exercise, they're best drunk post workout.

References

- The-athletes-nutrition-needs, sports-nutrition: nestle.com.au, Retrieved 2 March, 2019
- Sports-supplements, teens, en: kidshealth.org, Retrieved 3 April, 2019
- Sports-drink, medicine-and-dentistry, topics: sciencedirect.com, Retrieved 4 May, 2019
- Sports-drinks, lexicon: unesda.eu, Retrieved 5 June, 2019
- Sports-drinks-vs-water, sports-drinks-energy-drinks-and-soft-drinks, food-and-drink: choice.com.au, Retrieved 6 July, 2019
- Difference-between-hypotonic-isotonic-and-hypertonic-sports-drinks, fuel-better: veloforte.cc, Retrieved 7 August, 2019
- Hypertonic-drinks, lexicon: unesda.eu, Retrieved 8 January, 2019
- Difference-between-hypotonic-isotonic-and-hypertonic-sports-drinks, fuel-better: veloforte.cc, Retrieved 9 February, 2019

Physical Therapy and Rehabilitation

CHAPTER 5

Physical therapy is a type of physical rehabilitation which uses evidence-based kinesiology, exercise prescription, joint mobilization, electrotherapy and health education to treat the conditions such as soft tissue injuries, arthritis, etc. Rehabilitation seeks to restore functional ability to those with physical impairments or disabilities. The chapter closely examines the key concepts of physical therapy and rehabilitation to provide an extensive understanding of the subject.

PHYSICAL THERAPY

Physical therapy helps people of all ages who have medical conditions, illnesses or injuries that limit their regular ability to move and function.

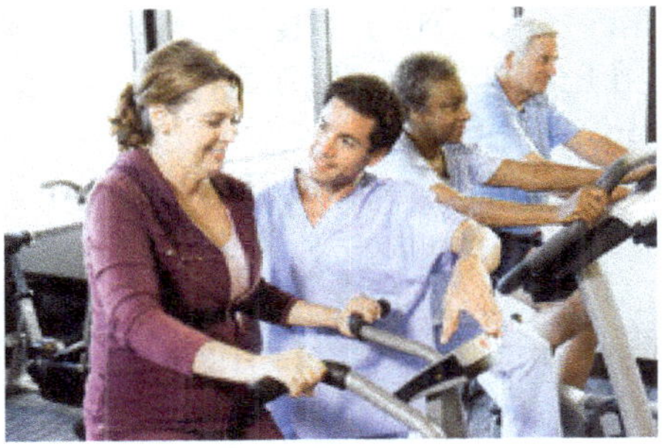

A customized physical therapy program can help individuals return to their prior level of functioning, and encourage activities and lifestyle changes that can help prevent further injury and improve overall health and well being. Primary care doctors often refer patients to physical therapy at the first sign of a problem, since it is considered a conservative approach to managing problems.

1. Reduce or eliminate pain: Therapeutic exercises and manual therapy techniques such as joint and soft tissue mobilization or treatments such as ultrasound, taping or electrical stimulation can help relieve pain and restore muscle and joint function to reduce pain. Such therapies can also prevent pain from returning.
2. Avoid surgery: If physical therapy helps you eliminate pain or heal from an injury, surgery may not be needed. And even if surgery is required, you may benefit

from pre-surgery physical therapy. If you are going into a surgery stronger and in better shape, you will recover faster afterwards in many cases. Also, by avoiding surgery, health care costs are reduced.

3. Improve mobility: If you're having trouble standing, walking or moving—no matter your age—physical therapy can help. Stretching and strengthening exercises help restore your ability to move. Physical therapists can properly fit individuals with a cane, crutches or any other assistive device, or assess for orthotic prescription. By customizing an individual care plan, whatever activity that is important to an individual's life can be practiced and adapted to ensure maximal performance and safety.

4. Recover from a stroke: It's common to lose some degree of function and movement after stroke. Physical therapy helps strengthen weakened parts of the body and improve gait and balance. Physical therapists can also improve stroke patients' ability to transfer and move around in bed so that they can be more independent around the home, and reduce their burden of care for toileting, bathing, dressing and other activities of daily living.

5. Recover from or prevent a sports injury: Physical therapists understand how different sports can increase your risk for specific types of injuries (such as stress fractures for distance runners). They can design appropriate recovery or prevention exercise programs for you to ensure a safe return to your sport.

6. Improve your balance and prevent falls: When you begin physical therapy, you will get screened for fall risk. If you're at high risk for falls, therapists will provide exercises that safely and carefully challenge your balance as a way to mimic real-life situations. Therapists also help you with exercises to improve coordination and assistive devices to help with safer walking. When the balance problem is caused by a problem in one's vestibular system, Physical therapists can perform specific maneuvers that can quickly restore proper vestibular functioning, and reduce and eliminate symptoms of dizziness or vertigo.

7. Manage diabetes and vascular conditions: As part of an overall diabetes management plan, exercise can help effectively control blood sugar. Additionally, people with diabetes may have problems with sensation in their feet and legs. Physical therapists can help provide and educate these patients on proper foot care to prevent further problems down the road.

8. Manage age-related issues: As individuals age, they may develop arthritis or osteoporosis or need a joint replacement. Physical therapists are experts in helping patients recover from joint replacement, and manage arthritic or osteoporotic conditions conservatively.

9. Manage heart and lung disease: While patients may complete cardiac rehabilitation after a heart attack or procedure, you also may receive physical therapy

if your daily functioning is affected. For pulmonary problems, physical therapy can improve quality of life through strengthening, conditioning and breathing exercises, and help patients clear fluid in the lungs.

10. Manage Women's Health and other conditions: Women have specific health concerns, such as with pregnancy and post-partum care. Physical therapists can offer specialized management of issues related to women's health. Additionally, PT can provide specialized treatment for: Bowel incontinence, breast cancer, constipation, fibromyalgia, lymphedema, male pelvic health, pelvic pain, and urinary incontinence.

If you have questions about how physical therapy may help you or someone you care about, please don't hesitate to ask your health care provider or local PT for information.

Different Types of Physical Therapy

Physical therapy can be a transformative experience, no matter when in life you take advantage of it. You might be surprised at the kind of impact that physical therapy can have; but it's a discipline that's been developed over many years, and physical therapists are able to help in many different ways, with many different challenges. Here's a breakdown of a few of them.

Pediatric Physical Therapy

Childhood is a time when the body grows very fast, and problems in childhood can have a negative effect on the rest of a person's life. Pediatric physical therapy is particularly designed to help adolescents, children and babies to make the most of their growth, overcome problems, and build their muscular and skeletal strength, often teaching them movement types and ranges of movement which they may never have experienced before.

Geriatric Physical Therapy

Getting older can be very tough on the muscles and skeleton. Over our lives, we can get used to using our muscles in ways which are unhealthy or unwise, such as bad posture or damaging gait, which we often don't recognize because we compensate for them using the rest of our bodies; but as we get older, we may notice more problems, as our muscles stop being strong enough to compensate as they have in the past. Geriatric physical therapy is about taking steps to use the muscles you have in a way which is more efficient and safe, and is less likely to lead to injuries.

Vestibular Rehabilitation

Balance feels like a tiny thing, until you don't have it any more. Vestibular rehabilitation focuses on helping you to overcome problems of the inner ear which can destroy your balance and be seriously debilitating, including chronic dizziness and vertigo. Physical therapy can help you to teach your body to have better balance and use its muscles to be steadier and sturdier.

Neurological Physical Therapy

Neurological problems, such as spinal cord injuries, strokes, multiple sclerosis, Parkinson's, Alzheimer's, brain injuries or cerebral palsy, strike at the nervous system, which is how your brain controls your body. Most neurological problems are chronic, meaning they are unlikely to be healed outright; but physical therapy can have a huge positive impact on life with a neurological disorder. By learning and practicing small therapeutic exercises, the effects of neurological disorders on muscles and movement can be smoothed off and made much more manageable.

Orthopedic Physical Therapy

Orthopedic physical therapy is designed to help you to recover muscle strength, as you might need to after an injury has left you unable to use certain muscles. Whether you've been injured recently and need to recover your strength after surgery, or you've been carrying an old injury for a long time, you may be surprised at the effect the precision, targeted exercises given to you by a physical therapist can have over time.

Cardiovascular/Pulmonary Physical Therapy

Cardiopulmonary physical therapy is about building independence if you have a serious cardiovascular or pulmonary problem – a problem with your heart or circulation. These problems could include heart attacks, or pulmonary fibrosis, and physical therapy can help you to grow strength in key muscles, and improve your endurance. In the long run, cardiopulmonary physical therapy is designed to help you build your independence.

REHABILITATION IN SPORT

Rehabilitation is the restoration of optimal form (anatomy) and function (physiology). It is a process designed to minimize the loss associated with acute injury or chronic disease, to promote recovery, and to maximize functional capacity, fitness and performance.

Musculoskeletal injuries are an inevitable result of sport participation. Football has the highest incidence of catastrophic injuries, with gymnastics and ice hockey close behind. Tissue injury from sports can be classified as macrotraumatic and microtraumatic.

- Macrotraumatic injuries are usually due to a strong force – such as a fall, accident, collision or laceration – and are more common in contact sports such as football and rugby. These injuries can be primary (due to direct tissue damage) or secondary (due to transmission of forces or release of inflammatory mediators and other cytokinesis).

- Microtraumatic injuries are chronic injuries that result from overuse of a structure such as a muscle, joint, ligament, or tendon. This type of injury is more common in sports such as swimming, cycling and rowing.

The process of rehabilitation should start as early as possible after an injury and form a continuum with other therapeutic interventions. It can also start before or immediately after surgery when an injury requires a surgical intervention.

Rehabilitation Plan

The rehabilitation plan must take into account the fact that the objective of the patient (the athlete) is to return to the same activity and environment in which the injury occurred. Functional capacity after rehabilitation should be the same, if not better, than before injury.

The ultimate goal of the rehabilitation process is to limit the extent of the injury, reduce or reverse the impairment and functional loss, and prevent, correct or eliminate altogether the disability.

Multidisciplinary Approach

The rehabilitation of the injured athlete is managed by a multidisciplinary team with a physician functioning as the leader and coordinator of care. The team includes, but is not limited to, sports physicians, physiatrists (rehabilitation medicine practitioners), orthopaedists, physiotherapists, rehabilitation workers, physical educators, coaches, athletic trainers, psychologists, and nutritionists. The rehabilitation team works closely with the athlete and the coach to establish the rehabilitation goals, to discuss the progress resulting from the various interventions, and to establish the time frame for the return of the athletes to training and competition.

Communication is a vital factor: A lack of communication between medical providers, strength and conditioning specialists, and team coaches can slow or prevent athletes from returning to peak capability and increase the risk of new injuries and even more devastating reinjuries.

Principles

Principles are the foundation upon which rehabilitation is based. Here are seven principles of rehabilitation, which can be remembered by the mnemonic (ATC IS IT):

- A: Avoid aggravation- It is important not to aggravate the injury during the rehabilitation process. Therapeutic exercise, if administered incorrectly or without good judgment, has the potential to exacerbate the injury, that is, make it worse.

- T: Timing- The therapeutic exercise portion of the rehabilitation program should begin as soon as possible—that is, as soon as it can occur without causing aggravation. The sooner patients can begin the exercise portion of the rehabilitation program, the sooner they can return to full activity. Following injury, rest is sometimes necessary, but too much rest can actually be detrimental to recovery.
- C: Compliance- Without a compliant patient, the rehabilitation program will not be successful. To ensure compliance, it is important to inform the patient of the content of the program and the expected course of rehabilitation.
- I: Individualization- Each person responds differently to an injury and to the subsequent rehabilitation program. Even though an injury may seem the same in type and severity as another, undetectable differences can change an individual's response to it. Individual physiological and chemical differences profoundly affect a patient's specific responses to an injury.
- S: Specific sequencing- A therapeutic exercise program should follow a specific sequence of events. This specific sequence is determined by the body's physiological healing response.
- I: Intensity- The intensity level of the therapeutic exercise program must challenge the patient and the injured area but at the same time must not cause aggravation. Knowing when to increase intensity without overtaxing the injury requires observation of the patient's response and consideration of the healing process.
- T: Total patient- It must be considered the total patient in the rehabilitation process. It is important for the unaffected areas of the body to stay finely tuned. This means keeping the cardiovascular system at a preinjury level and maintaining range of motion, strength, coordination, and muscle endurance of the uninjured limbs and joints. The whole body must be the focus of the rehabilitation program, not just the injured area. Providing the patient with a program to keep the uninvolved areas in peak condition, rather than just rehabilitating the injured area, will help to better prepare the patient physically and psychologically for when the injured area is completely rehabilitated.

Components

Regardless of the specifics of the injury, however, here are fundamental components that need to be included in all successful rehabilitation programs:

Pain Management

Medications are a mainstay of treatment in the injured athlete - both for their pain relief and healing properties. It is recommended that they need to be used judiciously with a distinct regard for the risks and side effects as well as the potential benefits, which include pain relief and early return to play. Therapeutic modalities play a small, but important, part in the rehabilitation of sports injuries. They may help to decrease pain and edema to allow an exercise-based rehabilitation programme to proceed. By understanding the physiological basis of these modalities, a safe and appropriate treatment choice can be made, but its effectiveness will ultimately depend upon the patient's individualized and subjective response to treatment.

Flexibility and Joint ROM

Injury or surgery can result in decreased joint ROM mainly due to fibrosis and wound contraction.

Besides that, it is common for post-injury flexibility to be diminished as a result of muscle spasm, inflammation, swelling and pain. In addition to impacting the injured area, this also affects the joints above and below the problem, and creates motor pattern issues. Flexibility training is an important component of rehabilitation in order to minimize the decrease in joint ROM. Also, a variety of stretching techniques can be used in improving range of motion, including PNF, ballistic stretching and static stretching.

Strength and Endurance

Injuries to the musculoskeletal system could result in skeletal muscle hypotrophy and weakness, loss of aerobic capacity and fatigability. During rehabilitation after a sports injury it is important to try to maintain cardiovascular endurance. Thus regular bicycling, one-legged bicycling or arm cycling, an exercise programme in a pool using a wet vest or general major muscle exercise programmes with relatively high intensity and short rest periods (circuit weight training) can be of major importance.

Proprioception and Coordination

Proprioception can be defined as 'a special type of sensitivity that informs about the sensations of the deep organs and of the relationship between muscles and joints'. Loss of proprioception occurs with injury to ligaments, tendons, or joints, and also with immobilization.Proprioceptive re-education has to get the muscular receptors working, in order to provide a rapid motor response. Restoration of proprioception is an important part of rehabilitation.The treatment has to be adapted to each individual, considering the type of ents required when the athlete returns to the field post-injury. The goal of function-based rehabilitation programmes is the return of the athlete to optimum athletic function. Optimal athletic function is the result of physiological motor activations creating specific biomechanical motions and positions using intact anatomical structures to generate forces and actions.

The use of Orthotics

The use of orthotic devices to support musculoskeletal function and the correction of muscle imbalances and inflexibility in uninjured areas should receive the attention of the rehabilitation team. Appropriate orthotic application will result in restraint forces that oppose an undesired motion. A complete orthotic prescription should include the patient's diagnosis, consider the type of footwear to be used, include the joints it encompasses and specify the desired biomechanical alignment, as well as the materials for fabrication. Communication with the orthotist,who will fabricate or fit the brace, is of utmost importance in order to obtain a good clinical result.

Psychology of Injury

Injury is more than physical; that is, the athlete must be psychologically ready for the demands of his or her sport. The most immediate emotional response at the point of injury is shock. It's degree may range from minor to significant, depending upon the severity of the injury. It is important to note that denial itself is an adaptive response that allows an individual to manage extreme emotional responses to situational stress. Many individuals assist athletes through the recovery process and can foster psychological readiness, but they can also identify those who are physically recovered but require more time or intervention to be fully prepared to return to competition. Thus, rehabilitation and recovery are not purely physical but also psychological.

Mental skills in sports are often viewed as part of an individual's personality and something that cannot be taught. Many physicians feel that injured athletes either have or do not have the mental toughness to progress through rehabilitation. Mental skills, however, can be learned. One example for this is to provide proper goal setting, which has very important role in sports rehabilitation, because they can enhance recovery from injury. Goal setting needs to be measurable and stated in behavioral terms. The research indicates that goals should be challenging and difficult, yet attainable. It is important for physicians to help them focus on short-term goals as a means to attain long-term goals. For example, to set daily and weekly goals in rehabilitation process which will end in long-term goal like returning to play after an injury. It is important for sports medicine physicians to assist patients in setting goals related to performance process rather than outcomes, such as returning to play.

Stages of Rehabilitation

Initial Stage of Rehabilitation

This phase lasts approximately 4-6 days. The body's first response to an injury is inflammation. It's main function is to defend the body against harmful substances, dispose of dead or dying tissue and to promote the renewal of normal tissue. The goals during the initial phase of the rehabilitation process include limitation of tissue damage, pain relief, control of the inflammatory response to injury, and protection of the affected anatomical area. The pathological events that take place immediately after the injury could lead to impairments such as muscle atrophy and weakness and limitation in the joint range of motion. These impairments result in functional losses, for example, inability to jump or lift an object. The extent of the functional loss may be influenced by the nature and timing of the therapeutic and rehabilitative intervention during the initial phase of the injury. If functional losses are severe or become permanent, the athlete now with a disability may be unable to participate in his/her sport.

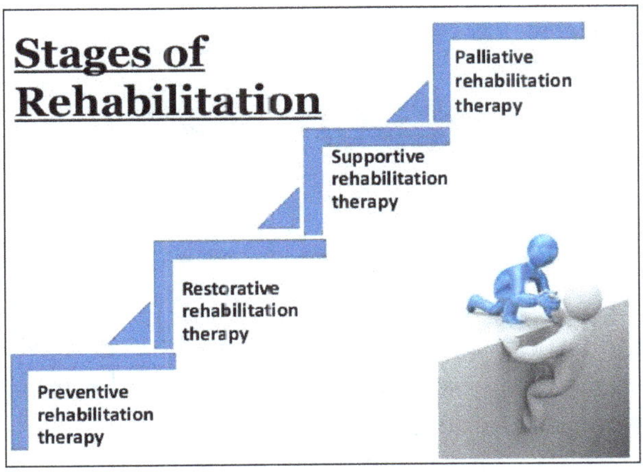

The physiotherapist is usually the professional in charge of this phase although the process may be started by a medical doctor.

Control Pain and Swelling

Primary treatment in initial phase of rehabilitation is RICE. It is the term that stands for Rest, Ice, Compression and Elevation. RICE can be used immediately and 24 to 48 hours after many muscle strains, ligament sprains, or other bruises and injuries.

Therapeutic modalities and medications are used to create an optimal environment for injury repair by limiting the inflammatory process and breaking the pain-spasm cycle. Use of any modality depends on the supervising physician's exercise prescription, as well as the injury site, and type and severity of injury. In some cases, a modality may be indicated and contraindicated for the same condition. For example, thermotherapy (heat therapy) may be contraindicated for tendinitis during the initial phase of the exercise program. However, once acute inflammation is controlled, heat therapy may be indicated. Frequent evaluation of the individual's progress is necessary to ensure that the appropriate modality is being used.

Despite the fact that rapid return to competition is crucial, rest is necessary to protect the damaged tissue from additional injury. Therefore, exercise involving the injured area is not recomended during this phase, although there are a few exceptions such as the tendinopathy protocols used to rehabilitate Achilles and patella tendon injuries. However, it is important to realize that a quick return to function relies on the health of other body tissues.

The power, strength, and endurance of the musculoskeletal tissues and the function of the cardiorespiratory system must be maintained. Athlete needs to understands the reasons for following a particular treatment regime or exercise program, as well medical professional's advice should be sought before embarking on any regime as more harm can be done than good if carried out incorrectly.

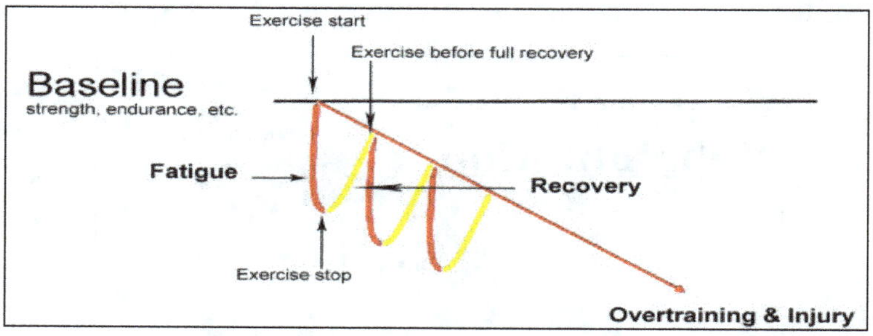

During the Recovery Phase.

Active range of motion is performed under one's own control, while passive range of motion occurs when another person or device produces the movement. If movement of the injured limb is not contraindicated, isolated exercises that target areas proximal and distal to the injured area may be permissible provided that they do not stress the injured area. Examples include hip abduction and rotation exercises following knee injury or scapula stabilizing exercises following glenohumeral joint injury. Isometric exercises are used for strengthening when range of motion is restricted or needs to be avoided due to the fracture or acute inflammation of a joint. Otherwise, isotonic strengthening can begin within the painless arc of joint motion.

Intermediate Stage of Rehabilitation

This phase lasts from day 5 to 8-10 weeks. After the inflammatory phase, the body begins to repair the damaged tissue with similar tissue, but the resiliency of the new tissue is low. Repair of the weakened injury site can take up to eight weeks if the proper amount of restorative stress is applied, or longer if too much or too little stress is applied.

Joint ROM and Muscle Conditioning

The goals during the second phase of rehabilitation include the limitation of the impairment and the recovery from the functional losses. Early protected motion hastens the optimal alignment of collagen fibers and promotes improved tissue mobility. A number of physical modalities are used to enhance tissue healing. Exercise to regain flexibility, strength, endurance, balance, and coordination become the central component of the intervention. To the extent that these impairments and functional losses were minimized by early intervention, progress in this phase can be accelerated. Again, the maintenance of muscular and cardiorespiratory function remains essential for the uninjured areas of the body. The strength and conditioning professional has considerable expertise to offer the other members of the sports medicine team regarding selection of the appropriate activities.

Possible exercise forms during this phase include strengthening of the uninjured extremities and areas proximal and distal to the injury, aerobic and anaerobic exercise, and improving strength and neuromuscular control of the involved areas:

- Isometric exercise may be performed provided that it is pain free and otherwise indicated. Submaximal isometric exercise allows the athlete to maintain neuromuscular function and improve strength with movements performed at an intensity low enough that the newly formed collagen fibers are not disrupted.
- Isokinetic exercise can be an important aspect of strengthening following injury. This type of exercise uses equipment that provides resistance to movement at a given speed (e.g., 60°/s or 120°/s).
- Isotonic exercise involves movements with constant external resistance and the amount of force required to move the resistance varies, depending primarily on joint angle and the length of each agonist muscle. Isotonic exercise uses several different forms of resistance, including gravity (i.e., exercises performed without equipment, with gravitational effects as the only source of resistance), dumbbells, barbells, and weight-stack machines. The speed at which the movement occurs is controlled by the athlete; movement speed can be a program design variable, with more acute injuries calling for slower movement and the later phases of healing amenable to faster, more sport-specific movement.
- Specific types of exercises exist to improve neuromuscular control following injury and can be manipulated through alterations in surface stability, vision, and speed. Mini-trampolines, balance boards, and stability balls can be used to create unstable surfaces for upper and lower extremity training. Athletes can perform common activities such as squats and push-ups on uneven surfaces to improve neuromuscular control.
- Exercises may also be performed with eyes closed, thus removing visual input, to further challenge balance.

Finally, increasing the speed at which exercises are performed provides additional challenges to the system. Specifically controlling these variables within a controlled environment will allow the athlete to progress to more challenging exercises in the next stage of healing.

Advanced Stage of Rehabilitation

This phase begins at around 21 days and can continue for 6-12 months. The outcome of the previous phase is the replacement of damaged tissue with collagen fibers. After those fibers are laid down, the body can begin to remodel and strengthen the new tissue, allowing the athlete to gradually return to full activity. This phase of rehabilitation represents the start of the conditioning process needed to return to sports training and competition. Understanding the demands of the particular sport becomes essential as well as communication with the coach. This phase also represents an opportunity to identify and correct risk factors, thus reducing the possibility of re-injury.

Functional Training

The combination of clinic-based and sport-specific functional techniques will provide an individualized, sport-specific rehabilitation protocol for the athlete. Rehabilitation and reconditioning exercises must be functional to facilitate a return to competition. Examples of functional training include joint angle-specific strengthening, velocity-specific muscle activity, closed kinetic chain exercises, and exercises designed to further enhance neuromuscular control. Strengthening should transition from general exercises to sport-specific exercises designed to replicate movements common in given sports. Cross-training is encouraged, especially with activities that do not produce any symptoms from the injury.

It is essential that the rehabilitation and training be sufficiently vigorous to prepare the injured tissue for the demands of the game. With each increase in activity, signs of recurring pain or weakness should trigger a slowdown or a reversal to a tolerable level of activity. The player will have returned to game during this phase and will have ceased physiotherapy or individual rehabilitation while this process is still continuing. Unrestricted sports activity is not allowed until all of these steps have been completed and full-effort sports-specific activity is tolerated without symptoms.

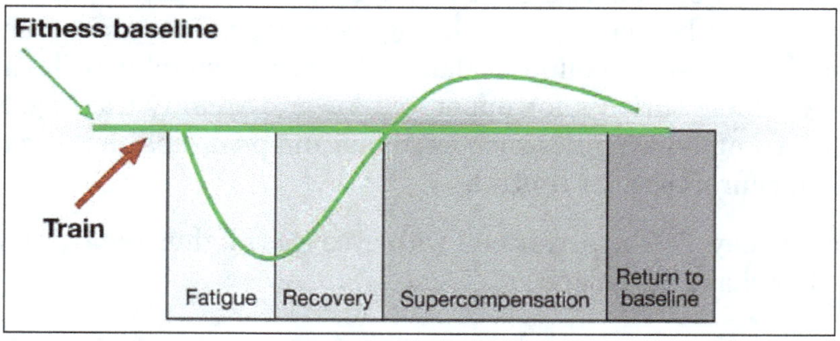

Adaptation Phase.

Return to Sport

At some point in the recovery process, athletes return to strength and conditioning programs and resume sport-specific activities in preparation for return to play. The transition is important for several reasons. First, although the athlete may have recovered in medical terms (ie, improvements in flexibility, range of motion, functional strength, pain, neuromuscular control, inflammation), preparation for competition requires the restoration of strength, power, speed, agility, and endurance at levels exhibited in sport.

Return to play is defined as the process of deciding when an injured or ill athlete may safely return to practice or competition. Early return to training and sport are considered sensible goals if the rate of return is based on the affected muscle, the severity of the injury and the position of the athlete.

Criteria for return to play must emphasize gradual return to sport-specific functional progressions. Sport-specific function occurs when the activations, motions and resultant forces are specific and efficient for the needs of that sport. Sport-specific functional rehabilitation should focus on restoration of the injured athlete's ability to have sport-specific physiology and biomechanics to interact optimally with the sport-specific demands. That means that they need to be replicated at the same speed, on the same surface and with the same level of fatigue to be truly effective.

Once a athlete has been medically cleared to return-to-play there are some fundamental steps that need to be followed:

- The athlete has to fulfill the fitness standards of the team he is returning to.
- The athlete needs to pass some skill specific tests applicable to his playing position.
- The player may then begin practicing with the team.
- Exposure to the match situation should be gradual, with the match time gradually increasing.

There are simple guidelines which need to be developed by each team with contributions and support from each member of the medical team.

Monitoring

Monitoring athlete well-being is essential to guide training and to detect any progression towards negative health outcomes and associated poor performance. Objective (performance, physiological, biochemical) and subjective measures (mood disturbance, perceived stress and recovery and symptoms of stress) are all options for athlete monitoring. Appropriate load monitoring can aid in determining whether an athlete is adapting to a training program and in minimizing the risk of developing non-functional overreaching, illness, and/or injury.

In order to gain an understanding of the training load and its effect on the athlete, a number of potential markers are available for use. There are a number of external load quantifying and monitoring tools, such as power output measuring devices, time-motion analysis, as well as internal load unit measures, including perception of effort, heart rate, blood lactate, and training impulse. Other monitoring tools used by high-performance programs include heart rate recovery, neuromuscular function, biochemical/hormonal/immunological assessments, questionnaires and diaries, psychomotor speed, and sleep quality and quantity. Coaching staffs and administrative personnel must work to ensure that care can be provided at all points of the rehabilitation process, especially when funding dictates the need to hire personnel capable of addressing injuries at multiple levels. A clear understanding of the injury and of the interventions from each provider is vital to an efficient and successful return to play.

Appropriate monitoring of training load can provide important information to athletes and coaches; however, monitoring systems should be intuitive, provide efficient data analysis and interpretation, and enable efficient reporting of simple, yet scientifically valid, feedback. If accurate and easy-to-interpret feedback is provided to the athlete and coach, load monitoring can result in enhanced knowledge of training responses, aid in the design of training programs, provide a further avenue for communication between support staff and athletes and coaches and ultimately enhance an athlete's performance.

THERAPEUTIC EXERCISE

Therapeutic exercises are specific solutions for physical therapy that are designed to treat particular problems like injuries, reduction in muscular function, impairment of skeletal function, minimized flexibility, and lack of strength and endurance by targeting them specifically. Because therapeutic exercises are specifically targeted to resolve a certain problem, it is not advisable to try them out on your own, and it's best to consult with a physical therapist if you have any issue that you would like to address with therapeutic exercises.

Types of Therapeutic Exercises

Therapeutic exercises are can be broadly grouped into the following categories:

Endurance exercises – These exercises are aimed at strengthening the muscles and improving your endurance by engaging the large muscle groups in your body. Endurance training only yields results when performed consistently for a considerable period of time, and are likely to need you to have a well-established level of strength before you start.

Strengthening exercises – These movements are performed with a greater resistance and fewer repetitions. Strengthening exercises improve the muscle power and strength when an accident or a surgery leaves a patient weaker; they take less time but need more energy than endurance exercises.

Flexibility exercises – These exercises come in handy when a patient has lost partial mobility of the arms or legs. By employing techniques like stretching, they improve the range of motion and mobilization. They tend to be small movements or gentle stretches, which can be surprisingly hard work, since they targeted at very specific muscle groups which have not been used for some time.

Balance and coordination exercises – These exercises help patients to maintain their center of gravity, and help improve balance and posture, making coordination easier in cases when this ability has been lost. They tend to require a lot of concentration to start with.

Benefits of Therapeutic Exercises

Therapeutic exercises aim to give various benefits to athletes, people who have recently had surgery, people who have had an accident that restricts movement, and anyone who has issues with musculoskeletal functions. These benefits could include:

Recovery from the effects of a stroke: One of the common aftermaths of a stroke is reduced movement in your limbs or extremities. These types of exercises can help you to regain strength and improve flexibility in the parts affected.

Recovery from sports-related injuries: Injuries sustained during sports and other heavy-duty physical activities can be treated using exercises. Physical therapy can also be used to prevent injuries in sportspeople.

Reduction or elimination of pain: therapeutic exercises can also be used to help treat achy joints and painful muscles. Manual therapy techniques like soft tissue and joint mobilization can help relieve stiffness and pain and keep aches from returning.

Managing lung and heart disease: therapeutic exercise can also help people with cardiac and pulmonary problems. By focusing on conditioning, strengthening, and breathing, these exercises help improve the quality of life in people with lung or heart disease.

Therapeutic Activity

Many times rehabilitation services are very necessary to improve the person's mobility and muscle strength. Through the use of therapeutic activity or therapeutic exercises (which are two very common activities), many physical therapists use these two interventions used to treat injury and dysfunction caused by disease.

Often times, physical therapy will conduct a thorough analysis of each individual patient and their physical capabilities. Usually, the physical therapist will then use their knowledge to correctly assess and shape a treatment plan that contains an appropriate exercise program that is highly customized for each unique patient. For example, often many older people suffer from hip fractures. Many times, this will cause issues with not only muscle strength but also mobility since it's such a difficult injury. In this case, a physical therapist will often prescribe therapeutic exercises in conjunction with therapeutic activities.

Goals of Therapeutic Activity

One of the first goals of a physical therapy exercise program is to help reduce pain and inflammation. After this is achieved, the exercise program can then focus on rebuilding and regaining muscle strength and mobility.

Therapeutic activity can also help with correcting faulty posture, inducing relaxation, and improving the overall levels of fitness in the body. This is why therapeutic exercises are often prescribed in addition to surgery, or in some cases, instead of surgery. All in all, these exercises, when done in the right way with a physical therapist, can offer remarkable benefits. If you think they might help, reach out to your physical therapist to talk through how therapeutic exercises could be good for you.

Choosing the Best Exercises for you

How do you know the best exercises which are specific to your condition? A good physical therapist will be able to accurately assess your condition and prescribe the right therapeutic exercise for your specific conditions. The grand majority of the exercises that your physical therapist will prescribe you will be very important for the success of your rehabilitation so make sure you find the time to do the exercises diligently. One suggestion is to facilitate a better recovery process is to proactively ask your physical therapist why he or she thinks the exercises they are recommending will help your specific condition or injury. This will also help you understand exactly why it's important to do the exercises.

PRINCIPLES OF EXERCISE AND SPORT TRAINING

When you approach your multisport training, the best way to answer your questions is to better understand the principles behind the work you are putting in to improve. These are seven basic principles of exercise or sport training you will want to keep in mind:

Individuality

Everyone is different and responds differently to training. Some people are able to handle higher volumes of training while others may respond better to higher intensities. This is based on a combination of factors like genetic ability, predominance of muscle fiber types, other factors in your life, chronological or athletic age, and mental state.

Specificity

Improving your ability in a sport is very specific. If you want to be a great pitcher, running laps will help your overall conditioning but won't develop your skills at throwing or the power and muscular endurance required to throw a fastball fifty times in a game. Swimming will help improve your aerobic endurance but won't develop tissue resiliency and muscular endurance for your running legs.

Progression

To reach the roof of your ability, you have to climb the first flight of stairs before you can exit the 20th floor and stare out over the landscape. You can view this from both a technical skills standpoint as well as from an effort/distance standpoint. In order to swim the 500 freestyle, you need to be able to maintain your body position and breathing pattern well enough to complete the distance. In order to swim the 500 freestyle, you also need to build your muscular endurance well enough to repeat the necessary motions enough times to finish.

Overload

To increase strength and endurance, you need to add new resistance or time/intensity to your efforts. This principle works in concert with progression. To run a 10-kilometer race, athletes need to build up distance over repeated sessions in a reasonable manner in order to improve muscle adaptation as well as improve soft tissue strength/resiliency. Any demanding exercise attempted too soon risks injury. The same principle holds true for strength and power exercises.

Adaptation

Over time the body becomes accustomed to exercising at a given level. This adaptation results in improved efficiency, less effort and less muscle breakdown at that level. That is why the first time you ran two miles you were sore after, but now it's just a warm up for your main workout. This is why you need to change the stimulus via higher intensity or longer duration in order to continue improvements. The same holds true for adapting to lesser amounts of exercise.

Recovery

The body cannot repair itself without rest and time to recover. Both short periods like hours between multiple sessions in a day and longer periods like days or weeks to recover from a long season are necessary to ensure your body does not suffer from exhaustion or overuse injuries. Motivated athletes often neglect this. At the basic level, the more you train the more sleep your body needs, despite the adaptations you have made to said training.

Reversibility

If you discontinue application of a particular exercise like running five miles or bench pressing 150 pounds 10 times, you will lose the ability to successfully complete that exercise. Your muscles will atrophy and the cellular adaptations like increased capillaries (blood flow to the muscles) and mitochondria density will reverse. You can slow this rate of loss substantially by conducting a maintenance/reduced program of training during periods where life gets in the way, and is why just about all sports coaches ask their athletes to stay active in the offseason.

The principles of specificity, progression, overload, adaptation, and reversibility are why practicing frequently and consistently are so important if you want to improve your performance. Missed sessions cannot really be made up within the context of a single season. They are lost opportunities for improvement. Skipping your long ride on weekend A means you can't or shouldn't go as far as originally planned on weekend B (progression & overload). Skipping your Monday swim means your swimming skills and muscles won't be honed or stressed that day (specificity). Missing a week due to a vacation sets you back more than one week (adaptation and reversibility). Apply these principles to your training to get a better understanding of your body and how to achieve success.

EXERCISES TO RECOVER FROM A SPORTS HERNIA

A sports hernia refers to a muscle or tendon injury in your lower abdominal or groin region. It's a painful injury frequently affecting athletes in sports that require frequent changes of direction, such as football, soccer, basketball and hockey.

The term "sports hernia" is a bit misleading. Unlike a regular hernia, the intestines do not poke through the abdominal wall. Put simply, a sports hernia can be considered an injury to your core muscle.

Banded Hip Flexion

How to: Attach a resistance band to a fixed object, lie down on the ground and wrap it around your left foot. Position yourself so there's tension in the band. With your core tight and feet dorsiflexed, bend your left knee and hip until both joints are at a 90-degree angle. Slowly straighten your leg to return to the starting position.

Sets/Reps: 2-3x6-8 each leg.

Physioball Dead Bug

How to: Lie on your back with your arms and legs straight over your shoulders and hips, respectively, and hold a physioball between your hands and feet. Keeping your core tight, simultaneously extend your left arm and right leg. Return your arm and leg to the physioball, and repeat with your opposite arm and leg. Continue alternating back and forth.

Sets/Reps: 2-3x6-8 each leg.

Glute Bridge Leg Lifts

How to: Lie on the ground with your knees bent and feet flat on the ground positioned about hip-width apart. Place a med ball between your knees and squeeze it with your legs. Drive your hips up as if performing a Glute Bridge. Tighten your core and glutes to create stability in this position. Without moving your hips, slowly straighten your left leg before returning it to the starting position. Repeat with your opposite leg and continue alternating back and forth.

Sets/Reps: 2-3x6-8 each leg.

CORE EXERCISES FOR ATHLETES TO BUILD STRENGTH AND FIGHT BACK PAIN

The core is a lot more than just the "six-pack." In fact the core consists of muscles from your chest down to your upper thighs, in every direction all around your body. Meanwhile, the muscle that causes the six-pack look is just one muscle, called the Rectus Abdominus. The rectus abdominus can flex the trunk just like you do when you perform Crunches and Sit-ups. That's why those exercises are so popular—they work this muscle, which gives you the "abs" look. The problem is that there are five other major muscle groups in the core that are just as—if not more—important to your spinal health and sports performance.

They are:

- External Obliques. These are the muscles that form the outer wall of your core along the sides. Like the rectus abdominus, they can help flex the trunk. They also help create rotation, so they're very involved with movements like throwing a baseball.
- Sitting just beneath the external obliques are the Internal Obliques. These muscles run from the pelvis up to the ribcage.
- Another major internal core muscle is the Transverse Abdominus, or "TVA." This muscle wraps around you like a corset, helping to improve your stability.
- The last two core muscles we'll talk about here are the Spinal Erectors in your back and the Hip Flexors, located on the front of your hips.

These two muscles can contribute to a common condition in athletes called anterior pelvic tilt, in which the pelvis dumps forward and tallbone hikes up behind them. A little anterior pelvic tilt is okay, but too much can be a bad thing. Good core workouts will help keep anterior pelvic tilt in check.

Most Core Exercises Get Wrong

Here's the problem with some of the most popular core exercises out there--moves like Sit-Ups, Crunches and Russian Twists. All of these moves, which require the spine to do a lot of bending or twisting, can be risky.

Why? Because those movements place an undo amount of stress on the spinal discs between each vertebrae. McGill's research shows that, with enough bends, those discs will suffer damage. It's not a question of "if." It's "when."

For this reason, McGill recommends that people ditch exercises that force you to do a lot of forward bending. His view is that you should save those bends for the times you really need them, like when you bend over to tie your cleats.

But there's another reason why traditional core exercises aren't all that effective for athletes: They ask the core to do a job that it's not really meant to do.

"The core is more of a force transmitter than a force producer," says Mike Robertson, co-owner of Indianapolis Fitness and Sports Training (IFAST) and physical preparation coach to the Indy Eleven professional soccer team. "It's not really meant to generate movement."

Most of the time, the muscles in your core are resisting motion, rather than creating it. A strong, stable core more shifts force from the lower body to the upper body by acting as a brace of sorts, transmitting energy from the ground to your outer extremities (the arms and legs).

"Athletes are not a collection of body parts. We need to unify our upper and lower bodies," explains Robertson. "Smart core training ties our upper and lower bodies together to help us create seamless and athletic movements."

Main Functions of Core Exercises

McGill's approach to core training does exactly what Robertson describes--ties the upper and lower body together with a strong, stable core. The movements he recommends train three functions of a healthy core:

- Anti-extension: This refers to exercises like Planks or Dead Bugs. When you perform these moves, the goal is for your core to prevent the lower back from arching. In biomechanics lingo, an "extended" lumbar spine is arched, while a "flexed" lumbar spine would be rounded. If you prevent your belly from sagging toward the ground while you hold a Plank, you are training anti-extension.
- Anti-rotation: This includes movements like the Pallof Press. In these exercises, you prevent your trunk from rotating against a sideways force.
- Anti-lateral flexion: Includes Side Planks and any exercise in which you're carrying an unbalanced load of heavy weights, such as a Contralateral Carry. In these movements, the goal is for your core to resist bending sideways. ("Lateral flexion" is the technical way to refer to a sideways bend).

While some of the 27 best core exercises for athletes will train one of these qualities solely, most hit several of these functions at once.

Best Core Exercises for Athletes

Taking into account everything we know about the core the many muscles it encompasses, how those muscles support the back, and how all of those tissues work with the spine to support you during sports, we've assembled this master list of 27 exercises. Every move on this list, performed correctly, will be safe for your spine. They can actually improve back pain in some instances.

They do not ask your spine to generate movement. By training your spine to perform in the way it was meant to perform, these exercises set you up for long term back health.

The exercises on this list are also more time efficient. Each of them trains your entire core--all of the major muscle groups we described above. You won't be wasting your time doing isolation moves that make you "feel the burn" for a few minutes but don't add much in terms of long-term value.

Finally, these exercises train your core to be strong and stable while your limbs are moving. This seems simple in theory, but in practice it's easy to let your midsection go soft when you move. That creates energy leaks and inefficient movements. By teaching your body how to brace while you move your arms and legs, you'll be more powerful in every sports movement you make.

RKC Plank

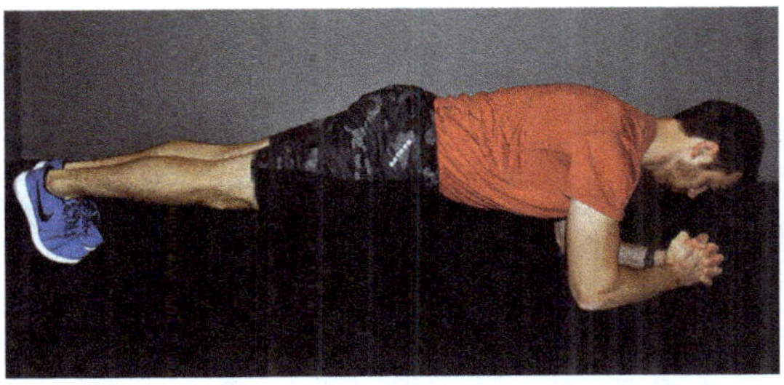

You simply need to hold your body in a straight line, which may look easy. And many of you may be able to hold a Plank for several minutes. But if you do it right, even the basic Plank should be incredibly challenging. The RKC Plank, which even the strongest athletes can hold for only 10-15 seconds.

How to:

- Assume a standard Plank position with your elbows under your shoulders, chin tucked and back straight.
- Squeeze your fists and lock in your shoulders by trying to rotate your arms outward.
- Squeeze your legs together and contract your quads and glutes.
- Imagine pulling your elbows to your toes as if moving into a pike position.

Mountain Climbers

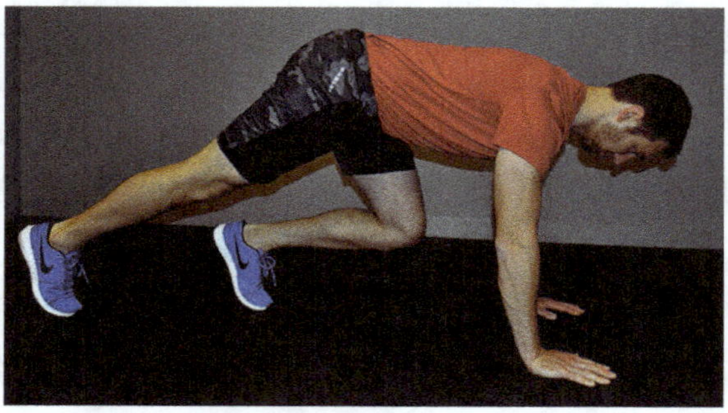

This popular exercise teaches your upper body to maintain its position during rapid leg movements, and can be used as an endurance move.

How to:

- Assume a push-up position with your back flat and core tight.
- Bring your right knee to your chest with your toes on the ground.
- Drive your right leg backward until it's straight and simultaneously bring your left knee to your chest.
- Continue bringing your knees to your chest in an alternating fashion. Do not bounce up and down.

Rolling Side Plank

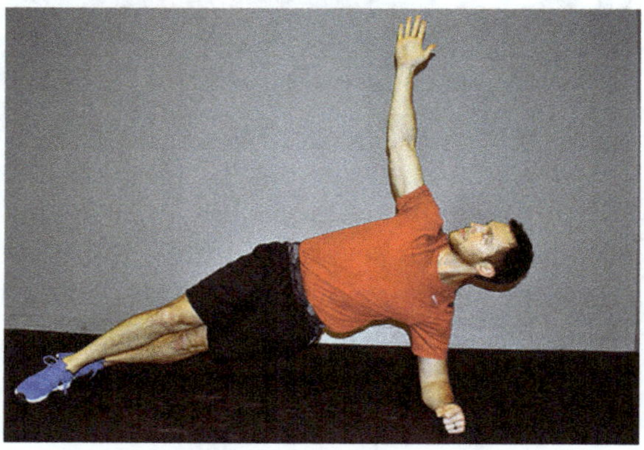

This combines a Plank and Side Plank, forcing your core muscles to brace during changing positions, making it challenging for both your abs and obliques.

How to:

- Lie on your side with your bottom elbow on the ground under eath your shoulder and your forearm perpendicular to your body.

- Position your top foot on the ground in front of your bottom foot. Raise your top arm vertically to form a T with your upper body.
- Drive your hips up to form a straight line with your body from head to toe. Tighten your abs, glutes and quads.
- Keeping your core tight, rotate your torso and place your opposite elbow on the ground to assume a Side Plank position on your opposite side.
- Continue slowly rolling side to side.

Physioball Circles

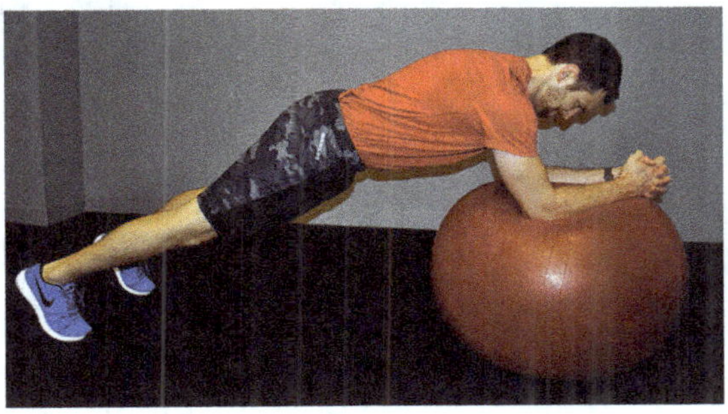

An advanced variation of the Plank, moving your forearms in a circle on a physioball makes the exercise unstable and your abs seriously burn.

How to:

- Assume a Plank position with your elbows on a physioball.
- Keeping your core tight, rotate your arms clockwise to move the physioball in a circle
- Repeat, moving your arms counterclockwise.

Physioball or TRX Pike to Rollout

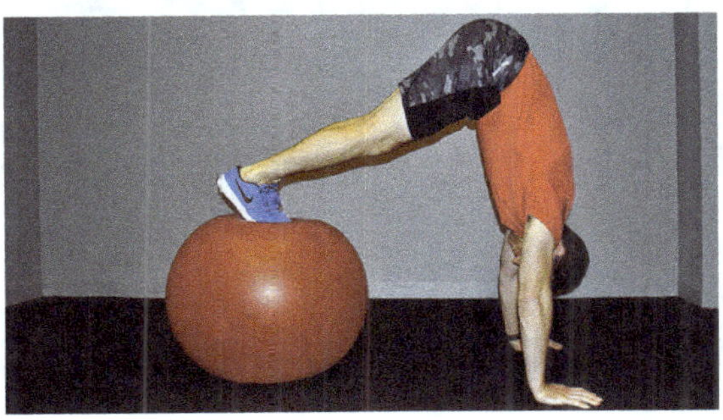

This may be the king of core exercises. It combines flexion and anti-extension moves to isolate the abs with minimal stress on the hip flexors and lower back.

How to:

- Assume a push-up position with your feet on a physioball. Keep your back straight and core tight.
- Drive your hips up so your body is in an inverted V position.
- Return to the starting position and drive your body back into a rollout.

Physioball Buzzsaw

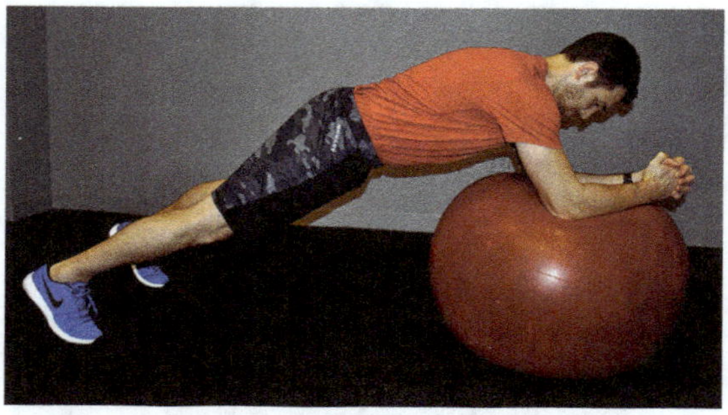

A great anti-extension core exercise that's more difficult than a Plank but easier than a Rollout, making this a great progression exercise.

How to:

- Assume a plank position with your elbows on a physioball.
- Keeping your core tight, drive your elbows forward to push the physioball forward.
- Roll the physioball back to the starting position.

Ab Wheel Rollout or Barbell Rollouts

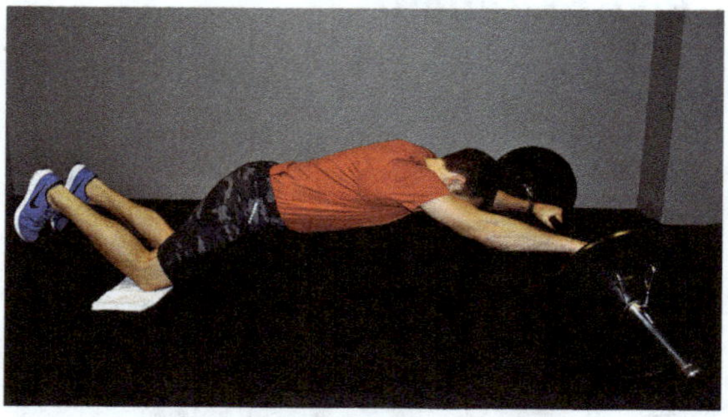

"[Your abs] don't bring your shoulders closer to your hips or your hips closer to your shoulders." "What they actually do is prevent you from going into extension." So, the Ab Wheel Rollout-which can also be done with a barbell-hits your abs better than any type of Crunch.

How to:

- Kneel on a towel or pad and grasp the ab wheel handles or barbell.
- Take a deep breath in and tighten your abs. Slowly roll forward until your arms are overhead and your torso is parallel to the floor.
- Keep your hips slightly elevated-don't drive them to the floor.
- Roll the wheel back toward your knees to return to the starting position.

Renegade Row

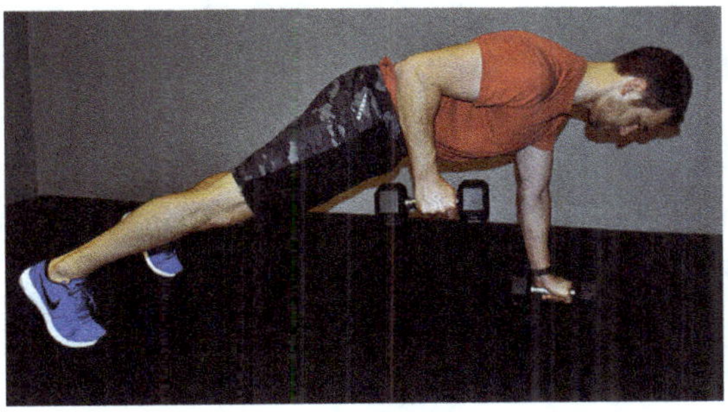

Everything in your core along with muscles in your shoulders, back, chest, hips and even quads have to work to keep you in the proper position during this exercise. "The Renegade Row is an indication that everything in your body is firing and firing proportionately," says Dr. Joel Seedman, owner of Advanced Human Performance. That's why it's the ultimate test of core strength.

How to:

- Set up two dumbbells parallel to each other about a foot apart.
- Assume a push-up position with your hands grasping the dumbbells instead of flat on the ground. Position your feet shoulder-width apart.
- Tighten your core and keep your back flat and hips square to the ground.
- Pick up the right dumbbell and row it to your side.
- Slowly lower the dumbbell and repeat. Perform on the opposite side.

Hanging Leg Raises

According to Brian Nguyen, owner of Brik Fitness and Mark Wahlberg's personal trainer, simply hanging on the bar is core work for the upper body. "Some of my favorite exercises to do for the core involve static shoulders and dynamic hips," he says. Add a Leg Raise, and your entire core works to produce movement while preventing your body from swinging back and forth.

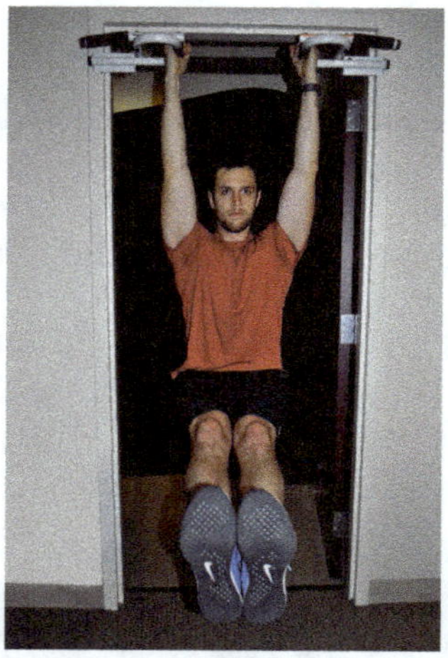

How to:

- Hold onto a bar as if performing a Pull-Up with your arms and legs straight.
- Keeping your core tight, bring your legs up until they're parallel to the ground.
- Slowly lower your legs to the starting position.
- Do your best to avoid rocking back and forth.

Single-Leg Lowering

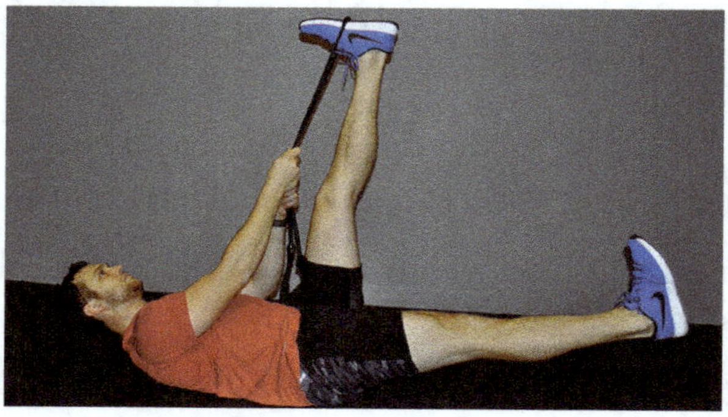

This is one of the most basic movements. Lots of athletes can perform it for many, many reps. But done right and paired with proper breathing technique, it's one of the best ways to activate your core muscles and restore your posture.

How to:

- Lie on your back and bring your left leg up until it's nearly perpendicular to the ground, depending on your flexibility. Wrap a resistance band around your left foot and hold it with your hands.
- Take a deep breath in.

- As you exhale, slowly lower your left leg and drive your heel away from you. Lower until your foot is a few inches above the ground.
- Inhale and raise your right leg up until it's next to your left leg.
- Repeat with your opposite leg.

Core-Engaged Dead Bug

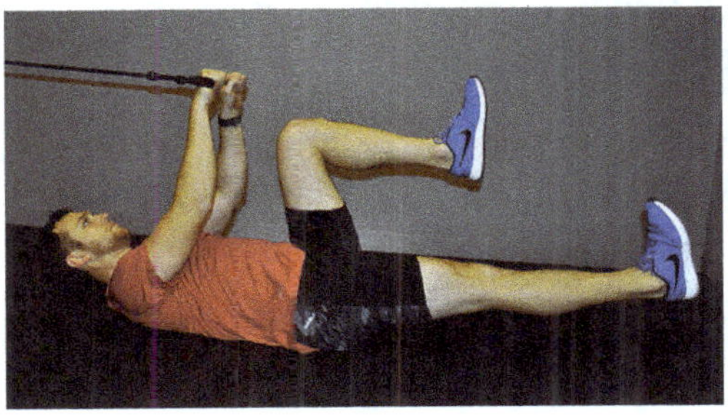

This exercise might look simple, but done right it's one of the best ways to train your core or prepare it for heavy training. The beauty of this exercise is that it improves breathing patterns and teaches your core to brace when your legs are moving, an essential skill for athletes.

How to:

- Lie on your back with your arms extended in front of your shoulders.
- Hold a resistance band or cable with the attachment or machine overhead.
- Bend your hips and knees to a 90-degree angle.
- Tighten your abs and press your lower back into the floor. Take a deep breath in.
- As you exhale, slowly extend your left leg toward the floor and bring your right arm overhead. Keep your abs tight and don't let your lower back arch.
- Slowly return your arm and leg to the starting position. Repeat with your opposite arm and leg.

The Lewit

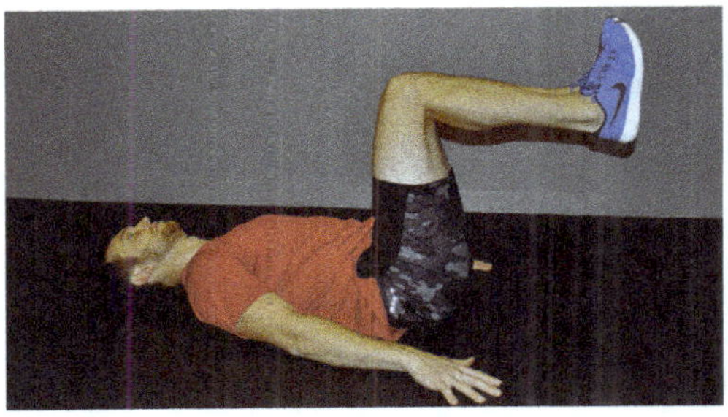

A corrective exercise, the Lewit engages your deep core muscles, which are difficult to develop with other movements.

How to:

- Lie on your back with your arms at your sides. Bend your hips and knees to a 90-degree angle. Maintain a naturally arched back.
- Slightly rock your pelvis forward and backward on your tailbone to fine-tune your back position.
- Once you're comfortable, take three normal breaths. Exhale normally on your third breath, then purse your lips and push any remaining air out of your lungs.
- Reset by rocking your pelvis and repeat the breathing pattern.

Turkish Get-up

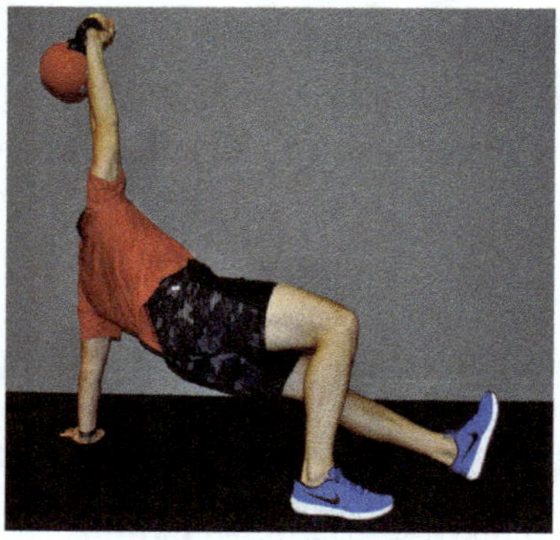

It looks weird and is tough to learn, but it's worth the trouble. According to Boyle, it's a fundamental movement that everyone should be able to perform. Plus, it builds serious core strength, improves mobility and increases shoulder stability.

How to:

- Lie on the ground holding a kettlebell in your right hand overhead.
- Bend your right knee and extend your opposite arm to the side. Fix your eyes on the kettlebell.
- Slowly sit up by shifting your weight to your left elbow and then your hand.
- Drive through your left hand and right heel to extend your hips and raise your body into a bridge position.
- Swing your left leg under your body and assume a kneeling position.
- Repeat on the other side.

Hollow Body Holds

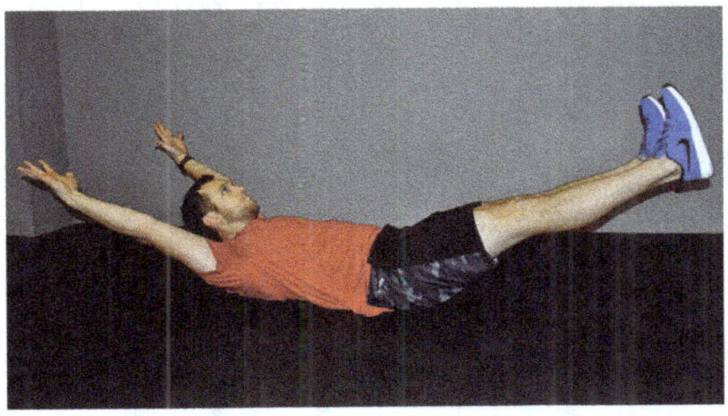

An exercise popular with gymnasts, this one strengthens the abs without wearing down the lumbar spine like a Crunch or Sit-Up.

How to:

- Raise your legs straight up, bring your arms overhead and crunch your shoulders up.
- Tighten your abs as if bracing for a punch, making sure your lower back is flat against the floor.
- Hold this position, making sure to breathe throughout the hold.

Modified Curl-up

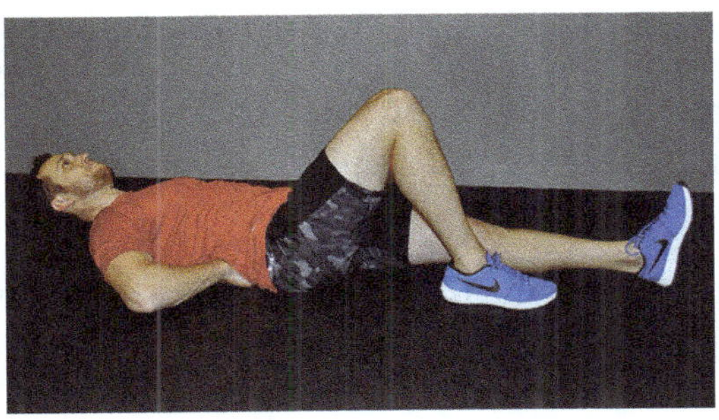

As a substitute for Crunches and Sit-Ups, Dr. Stuart McGill, a leading spine researcher at the University of Waterloo, recommends the Modified Curl-Up. It looks sort of like a Crunch, but the actual movement is significantly different and safe for the lumbar spine. "This Curl-Up is light years away from a standard abdominal crunch exercise," says McGill.

How to:

- Lie with your back on the floor.
- Place your hands flat under your lower back and raise your elbows slightly off the ground.
- Bend one leg so that your foot is in line with your opposite knee.

- Keeping a straight neck, tighten your abs as if bracing for a punch and raise your head and shoulders off the ground slightly. Hold this position for 10 seconds.
- Lower and repeat.

Reverse Crunch

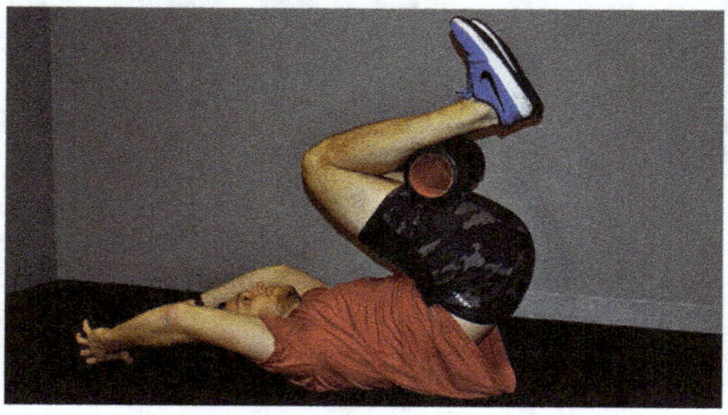

This is one of the best ways to directly target your abs, and it works. "It feels like you got kicked in the stomach a couple of times after you do them," says Dr. John Rusin, a strength coach and physical therapist.

How to:

- Lie back on a bench with your thighs perpendicular to the ground.
- Place a foam roller between your hamstrings and calves and squeeze the roller.
- Place your hands over your head and grab the sides of the bench.
- Forcefully contract your abs to lift your butt off the bench and your knees up above your chest. Hold this position for one or two seconds with a maximal ab contraction.
- Slowly lower back to the starting position until your butt is on the bench and your thighs are perpendicular to the ground.

Bird Dog

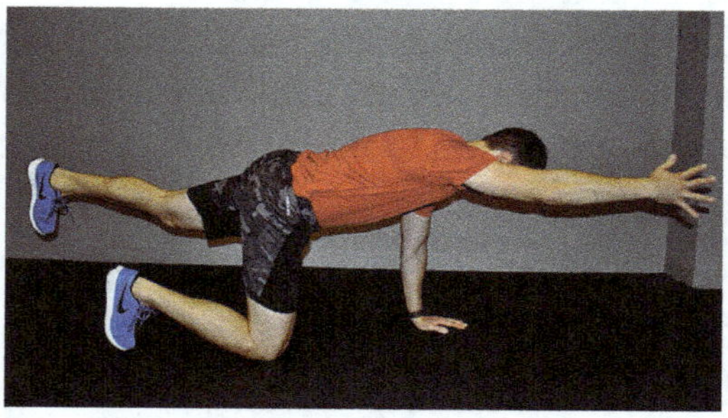

"Whether you're an athlete, bodybuilder, powerlifter, fitness enthusiast or an active individual looking for a way to improve your low-back function and spinal health, the

Bird Dog is a worthwhile drill that can enhance multiple aspects of performance and muscle function," says Dr. Seedman.

How to:

- While maintaining a flat back, kneel on the floor with your knees under your hips and your hands under your shoulders.
- Keeping your abs tight, raise your opposite arm and leg until they are straight and in line with your body. Do not arch your lower back.
- Return to the starting position and repeat with your opposite arm and leg.

Pallof Press

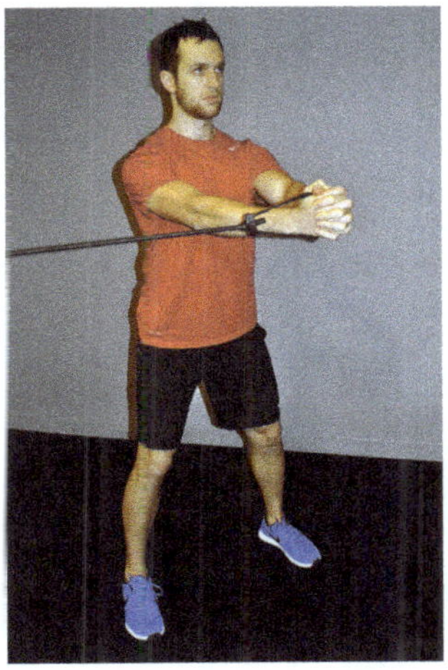

The Palloff Press trains your core to resist rotation. "A lot of times when we are working the core, we use things like super bands and do a lot of rotational work," says Todd Durkin. "Anti-rotation is great for stability of the obliques, core and lower back."

How to:

- Stand with your feet wider than hip width and position your body perpendicular to a cable machine.
- Grasp the cable handle with both hands directly in front of your chest.
- Keeping your core tight, extend your arms in front of your chest.
- Bring your hands back to your chest to return to the starting position.

Med Ball Rotational Throws

This one increases rotational power from your hips and core, which is critical for throwing a ball, swinging a bat or taking a slap shot.

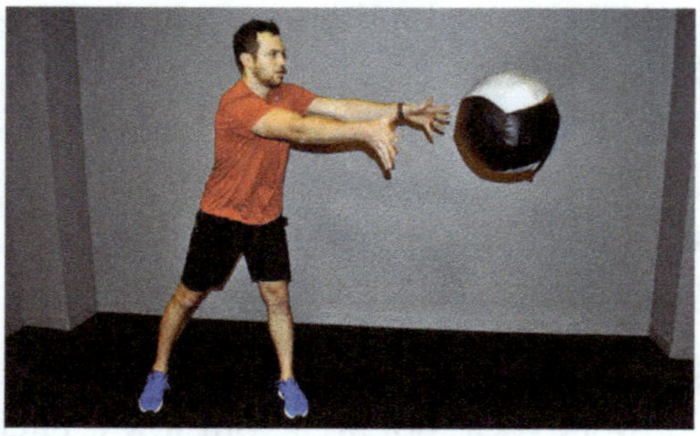

How to:

- Stand with your left side facing a wall about 5 feet away with your knees and hips bent, holding a med ball in front of your waist.
- Shift your weight to your right foot and swing the med ball to your right hip.
- Drive through your hips, rotate at your core and throw the med ball against the wall with an underhand toss.
- Catch the ball off the wall and immediately repeat.

Med Ball Slams

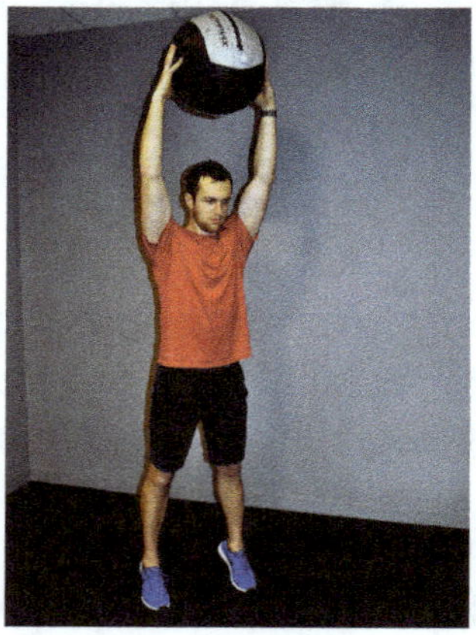

Increase your ability to explosively generate force through your lower body and core to power an upper-body movement.

How to:

- Stand with your feet hip-width apart holding a med ball at chest height with your arms extended.
- Rise up onto your toes, lift the med ball overhead and slam it straight down, generating power through your hips and core.
- Catch the ball off the bounce and set up for your next rep.

Farmer's Walks

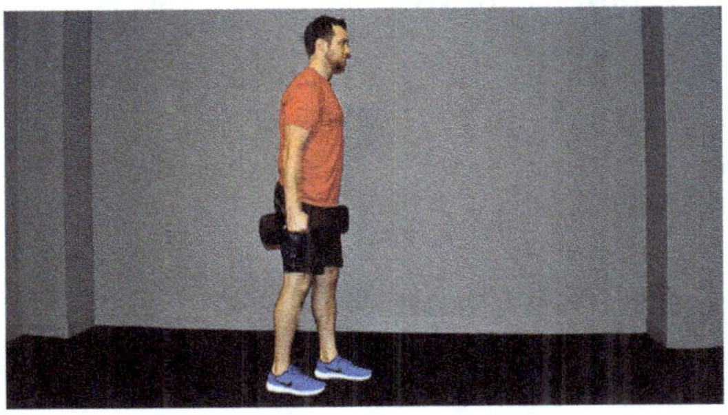

Once used primarily to increase grip strength, Farmer's Walks and other loaded carries are simply a moving Plank, where your core must fire to stabilize your trunk and hips while you walk with weight.

How to:

- Stand between two sets of weights—dumbbells, kettlebells or custom barbells—and grab hold of the weights.
- Brace your core and glutes and drive through the floor to lift the weights.
- Keeping your core tight, back flat and shoulders down and back, take small and quick steps for the allotted distance or time.
- Put the weights down carefully—do not simply drop them on the floor.

TRX Rip Trainer Pitchfork

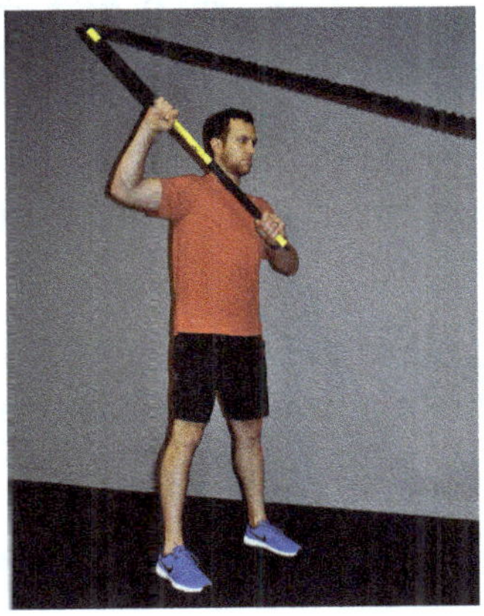

Pulling the Rip Trainer up and behind your body activates everything from your hands to your feet, while your core fights to prevent rotation and keep you upright.

How to:

- Assume a quarter-squat stance facing the cord mount.

- Hold the Rip Trainer in front with a shoulder-width, overhand grip; hold the bottom of the Rip Trainer with your left hand and your right hand near the cord.
- Simultaneously extend your hip and knees to drive the tip of the Rip Trainer over your shoulder. Briefly hold this position.
- Lower in control and repeat.

Wide-Stance Anti-Rotation Chop

A slow and controlled movement that teaches your core to produce and resist rotation through a full range of motion.

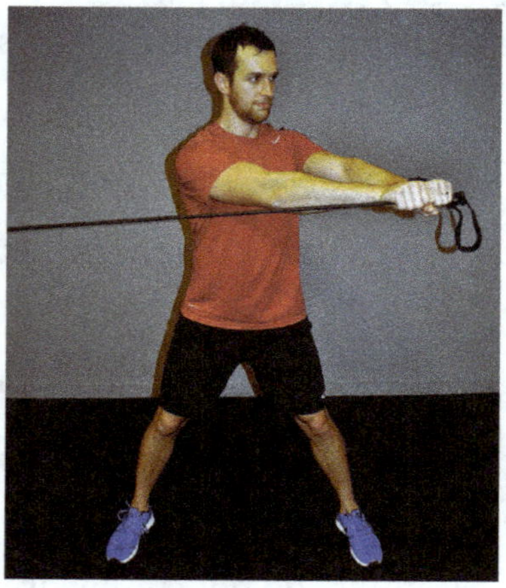

How to:

- Assume an extra-wide stance with a cable machine to your right.
- Hold the rope attachment in front of your chest with your arms extended.
- Rotate your upper body to the right as far as your range of motion allows without rotating through your lower back. Keep your arms directly in front of your chest—do not move your lower body.
- Reverse the movement and rotate your upper body toward the left as far as you can, pulling the rope attachment with you as you move.
- Continue rotating your torso in each direction.

Landmine Rainbow

"If you want a strong core that will help you perform athletically on the field, you need to perform integrated core exercises," says Tumminello. To do this, you need to work your core while engaging your shoulders and glutes.

"If you want a strong core that will help you perform athletically on the field, you need to perform integrated core exercises," says Tumminello. To do this, you need to work your core while engaging your shoulders and glutes.

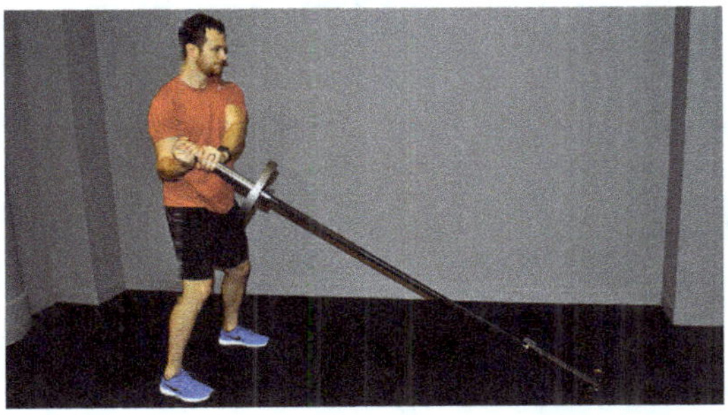

How to:

- Place a barbell in a landmine rack and load the desired amount of weight (it's best to start light).
- Stand directly in front of the end of the barbell and raise it above your head with both hands.
- While keeping your body stationary, move the barbell in a rainbow-like arc. Bend slightly at the elbows while moving the weight, but try not to rotate at the hips or shoulders.
- Stand tall throughout the movement.

Barbell Offset Iso Holds

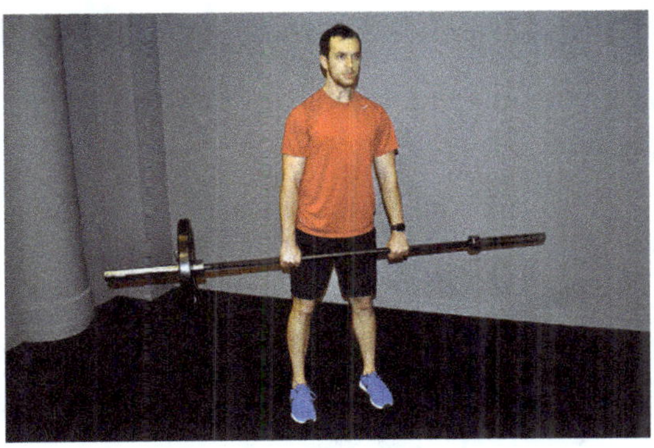

The uneven load on the barbell naturally pulls you to one side, and you have to tighten your entire core to maintain an upright position. "You are breathing and bracing under stress and really learning how to engage your core muscles, not just your six-pack muscles," says Matthew Ibrahim, strength coach and owner of Movement Resilience.

How to:

- Load a barbell with a plate on one side and position it on a rack at hip height.

- Grasp the bar with a shoulder-width grip and pick it up off the rack.
- Tighten your core as forcefully as possible for the specified duration before returning the bar to the rack.
- Complete your sets on one side, then switch the plate to the opposite side of the bar.

Contralateral Carries

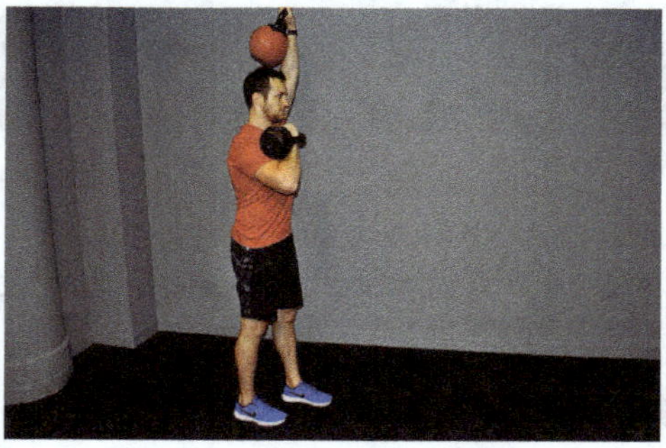

Holding a light kettlebell overhead and a heavy kettlebell in the rack position at your shoulder has benefits similars to Farmer's Walks, but it forces your core muscles to handle uneven loads in challenging positions.

How to:

- Hold a heavy kettlebell with your right hand at shoulder height in the rack position. Hold a lightweight kettlebell with your left hand overhead.
- Keep your core tight and back flat. Avoid arching through your lower back.
- Walk slowly for a specified distance or duration. Switch the positions of the kettlebells for the next set.

Heavy Lifts

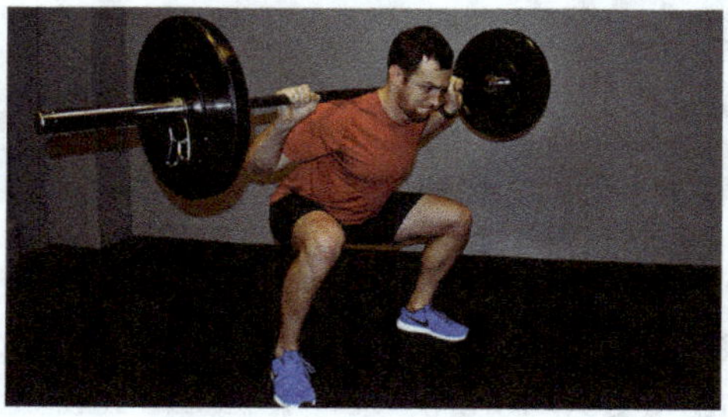

Squats, Deadlifts and their variations are among the best ways to develop a strong core. During the movement, your core muscles work overtime to keep your spine in place and handle the heavy weight load. Although they are effective, do not rely exclusively on heavy lifts to develop your core.

References

- Reasons-why-physical-therapy-is-beneficial: burke.org, Retrieved 10 March, 2019
- Different-types-of-physical-therapy: movementforlife.com, Retrieved 11 April, 2019
- Rehabilitation-in-Sportz: physio-pedia.com, Retrieved 12 May, 2019
- Therapeutic-exercise: movementforlife.com, Retrieved 13 June, 2019
- Principles-of-Exercise-and-Sport-Training, Multisport-Lab, USA-Triathlon: teamusa.org, Retrieved 14 July, 2019
- Exercises-to-recover-from-a-sports-hernia, a: stack.com, Retrieved 15 August, 2019
- Best-core-exercises?Splitctas=1, a: stack.com, Retrieved 16 January, 2019

Prevention of Sports Injuries

CHAPTER 6

Sports injury preventions are broadly classified into three categories: primary, secondary and tertiary prevention. Primary prevention involves the avoidance of injury, secondary prevention includes the early diagnosis and treatment of an injury, and tertiary prevention primarily focuses on the rehabilitation to reduce and correct an existing disability. This chapter discusses in detail the methods used to prevent injuries in various sports such as soccer and baseball.

Injuries are a serious problem in the training-competition process, since their occurrence leads to the modification or interruption of the activity. Any injury alters training plans and is an important factor in training monitoring. Within the sports community, the most common intervention focuses on recovering from injuries in order to return to previous performance levels; a process that is expensive from both the economic and sporting points of view. However, in many sports, strategies aimed at injury prevention have not been systematically implemented, despite their proven effectiveness. Some of preventive programs that must be incorporated in training schedules to minimize the impact of injuries. With regard to the introduction of intervention strategies in sport, through preventive measures from physical activity, it is necessary to review the power of the proposed measures and assess their effectiveness.

Multifactorial Analysis of the Model for Injury Prevention

One of the most important aspects of training and competition would be the control of the process and its development. The control of training comprehends all the aspects that permit the adaptation of the contents and the training load. One of the reasons why the modification of training programs becomes necessary is sports injuries, as they generate a partial or total interruption of the training process. It is a fact that is practically usual in the majority of sports, as a great number of sportsmen and women injury themselves at least once a season. The injuries constitute set-backs, which cannot be totally avoided, as the mere practice of sports carries with it the risk of injury happening. However, their impact could be lessened through the monitoring, controlling and analysing of the factors and their evolution by using adequate means of control.

The objective would be to ensure that the risk is lessened (prevention) or that its evolution is more favourable, and to ensure the incorporation of the sportsperson in as little time as possible (functional recuperation). Until a few years ago, efforts were centred on treating injure, paying special attention to the therapeutic process from a clinical perspective. However, in the last few years interest has become directed towards the development of strategies and multidisciplinary proposals related to the prevention of and the recovery from sports injuries. Therefore, the intervention performed presents a model of general control, which includes a global evaluation of the specific sporting context (sport, characteristics of the sportsperson, training conditions, etc.), an adequate prevention in the face of multiple factors of injury predisposition (multifactorial model), and a systematic effort in case of the injure appearing, guaranteeing a full recovery.

Sequence of Prevention

To establish a plan of prevention one must begin with Van Mechelen et al.´s proposal in a sequence of four steps: establishing the extent of the injury, identifying the factors and mechanisms of injury, introducing preventive measures and, lastly, evaluating their effectiveness. The last few decades have seen a significant increase in the epidemical studies contributing information on the first two steps: identifying injury incidence in each sport, along with the factors and mechanism involved in the production of the injuries, as well as establishing the possible factors provoking the injury, upon which to act in a preventive manner. To understand the importance of the problem it is necessary to know the injury profile for the different sports: injury frequency (number of injuries per 1,000 hours of training or competition), location of the different body structures, severity, typology and the rest of relevant aspects. developed a model to explain the different risk factors involved in producing sports injuries, rejecting approaches involving an only factor.

Model/ Stage	TRIPP (Finch,2006)	Van Mechelen et al.
1	Injury surveillance	Establishing extent of the problem
2	Establishing aetiology and mechanisms of injury	Establishing aetiology and mechanisms of injury
3	Developing preventive measures	Introducing preventive measures
4	“Ideal condition”/scientific evaluation	assessing their effectiveness by repeating stage1
5	Describing intervention context to inform implementation strategies	
6	Evaluating effectiveness of preventive measure in implementation context	

Later, this proposal is completed by showing the complex interaction of the internal and external risk factors and the mechanisms that cause sports injuries. In recent years, the theoretical framework of research has been expanded with contributions from Finch, increasing the number of steps in the sequence of prevention to the implementation and evaluation of injury prevention in a real context.

These injuries are associated to a series of risk factors that need to be identified so as to introduce preventive measures in training. This factors are classified in intrinsic factors (predisposal of the sportsperson) and extrinsic factors (exposal to factors of risk), although in reality the process indicates that these factors are produced in a complex manner and they interact between them.

Among the most important intrinsic factors would be the existence of a previous injury and inadequate rehabilitation, age, the sportsperson's state of health, psychological state and aspects, etc. With regard to extrinsic factors, these are: type of activity and motive gestures specific to the sport, dynamics of the training load, training and competition exposition time, material and equipment, type of surface of the playing, environmental conditions and anatomic fatigue.

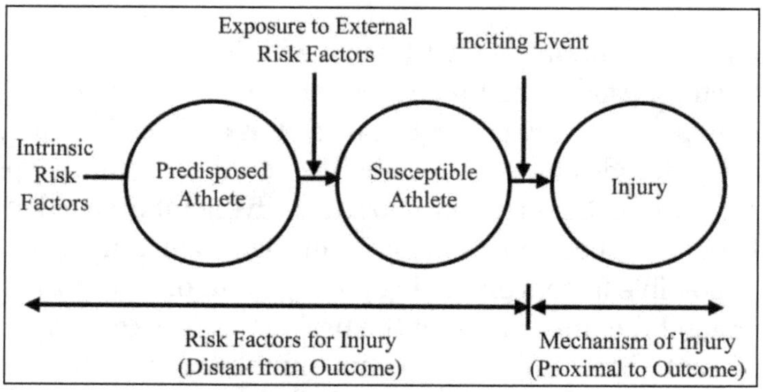

Recursive model of aetiology in sport injury.

Once the most frequent injuries of each modality and their risk factors are known, preventive measures can be introduced. The efficiency of these measures and their suitability from the methodological point of view are known beforehand. The prevention programs should be evaluated through more rigorous designs, with not only random experimental designs of group control, but also quasiexperimental designs that permit more representative samples (professional sportspeople) and more realistic practice contexts (training – competition processes), with truly ideal intervention programmes. Only in this way can the efficiency of the preventive intervention in sports be evaluated.

Different Levels of Sports Injury Prevention

Primary Level

The objective of the Primary Level of prevention is to avoid injury before it happens. It consists of a general preventive intervention taking into account the general factors and mechanisms characteristic of a given person and their effect on a sportsperson with an injury risk. This level implies a change in beliefs, attitude, habits and behaviour towards prevention, and their training by both coaches and sportspeople.

The main measures are of an indirect type: they will control the type, quality and state of the training grounds and competition surfaces; the type of footwear that respects cushioning, traction and rotation upon the field; the use of protective elements; the organization of travel; sleeping and eating habits; the use of tapping as a possible factor in reducing ligamentous affectations; or hydration, controlling the number and quantity of liquid intake and the combination with other sports drinks.

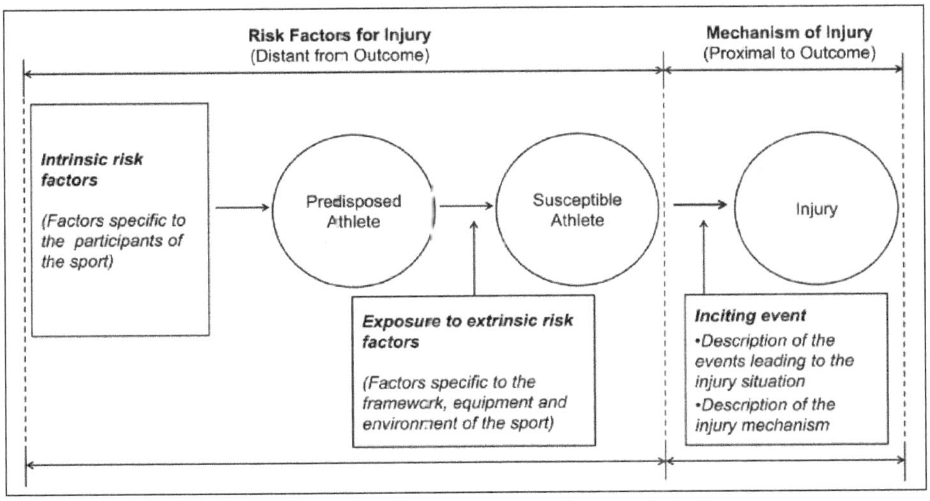

Factors related to the occurrence of sports injuries.

Secondary Level

The Secondary Level of prevention constitutes an early level of detection in which intervention takes place in the stages immediately previous to injury or when it has already happened. At this level, one must be in contact with the sportsperson in risk of injury with the objective of diagnosing and detecting the injury once it has occurred by means of the appearance of signs and symptoms. Through the analysis and the discovery of the different risk indicators, there is the possibility of intervening by organizing programmes of intervention at an individual or group level.

The tendency nowadays entails identifying risk values by means of an exhaustive process of evaluating and monitoring of the sportsperson. Clinical, physical and motor tests will be used to obtain risk indicators, as well as registering and analysing the clinical history of said sportsperson and his/her injuries in previous seasons. Age, competition experience, fatigue and overtraining will be taken into account with regard to exposal to training and competition, as well as psychological factors, reducing or controlling those situations which are potentially stressing for the sportsperson.

Tertiary Level

The Tertiary Level of prevention is the prediction and treatment of possible complications during the post-injure phase. This constitutes an individual level of prevention that involves reducing the grade of injury incidence by eliminating all those contents and work means that could worsen the injury or its consequences and executing programmes directed towards developing the elements of protection from a specific injury. The elements of intervention at this level should be directed towards regulating and reducing mechanical, muscular, articular, ligament or tendon imbalance that a sportsperson may be exposed to after a specific injury.

Basics of Preventive Measures through Physical Activity

Warm up

The efficiency of warm up in the training-competition process is explained by the change of the viscoelastic properties of tissues with increasing temperature or the improvement of metabolic conditions. Content such as joint mobility, jogging, stretching, and proprioceptive technical training prior to the main activity provide an important preventive security.

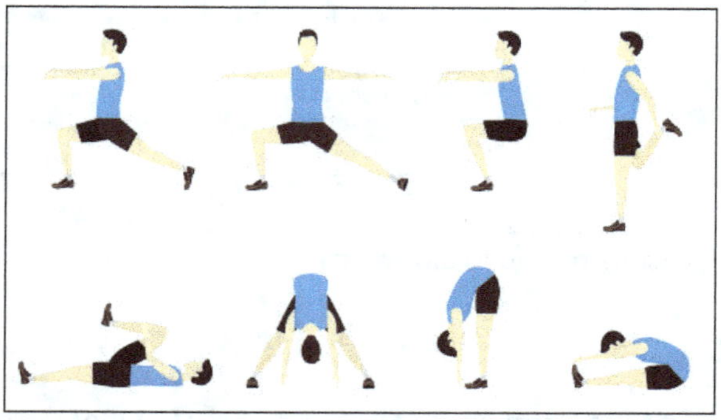

Examples of exercises with preventive content in warm-up.

Different studies have found a relation between the absence or deficient execution of warmup and posterior injury in specific actions of the sportand, in contrast, proposed tactics that introduce preventive contents, which include the previously mentioned elements, manage a decrease of the number of injuries.

Strength

Strength plays an important role in the stabilisation of different bodily structures through the normal functioning of passive stabilizers (articular: ligamental structures and meniscus) and active stabilizers (muscles), as well as the interaction between both. The bibliography argues the protective factor that muscle can provide by contributing active stability to the different articular structures, as well as the correct balance between the different muscular groups, developing a fixative and balancing function which allows the individual to develop specific actions with the greatest safety possible, without risk of injury. The main goal of working strength as a means of prevention is to ensure the correct balance between the different bodily structures, thus permitting the safe development of the different actions specific to each sport.

Right Artromuscular Balance as Preventive Tool

The practice of sports implies the practice of certain structures in a repetitive manner, which generates a muscular imbalance between antagonistic/agonistic groups.

Maintaining a correct artromuscular balance, permitting a lessening of the effects of muscle shortening and weakening, and maintaining the integrity of articulations would be the main preventive objective of strength work.

With this goal in mind, there are different evaluation measures, such as isokinetic appreciation, that can determinate the grade of functional balance between agonistic and antagonistic muscle. The main investigations about this topic establish a ratio that connects both values, fundamentally in the thigh muscle (hamstrings/quadriceps) whose incidence is related to muscle injure and a protective function of the knee articulation. Main investigations place adequate ratio values at the following reference values:

The value of functional ratio that discriminates the probability of injury is between 0.60 and 0.70 This same value is the one shown for an imbalance bearing a muscular recurrence.

Besides, recent investigations highlight the relationship between the balance of strength values between a dominant and non-dominant leg. It is established that a good balance should not exceed 10% between them, and in case of exceeding this percentage, the probability of injury would increase, and risk limit of bilateral asymmetry in the strength is at 15%.

In other muscle groups also involved in many sports, the normal ratios between agonist and antagonist muscles are in: adduction/abduction of hip, with hand-held dynamometer, between 0.96 and 1.4 depending on the rating, side lying position and supine position respectively; and, concentric isokinetic 60º/s-1 and 120º/s-1are between 0.68 and 0.76, also depending on the position in which the test is performed. Concerning the shoulder joint, the ratios measured with isokinetic vary depending on the sport practiced so for the rotation ratio internal / external rotation, 60º/s-1 and 120º/s-1, between 1 and 1.3, but can reach a value of 2 for specialists sports pitches, both team sports and individual sports; and, for adduction/abduction and extension/ flexion, normal values are 30% higher than for adduction to abduction, and 50% higher for extensors than for flexors. Functional jump tests are also used to determine possible asymmetries associated to bilateral strength deficits. The majority of them are taken from evaluations of the functional state of the lower extremity after anterior cruciate ligament (ACL) injury, and many studies show their usefulness. Although jump distance tests do not contribute with the sophisticated analysis of the working of the lower extremity that can be obtained from studies of running and strength platforms, jump tests seem useful as an evaluation of early detection that does not require a specialised equipment, it can be done in a short time and uses opposite extremity as control. The highly specific nature and low number of false positives makes these tests useful in confirming asymmetries of lower extremities. By associating them with other clinical evaluating tools, they confirm the magnitude of functional limitations.

It seems that both the progressive test (Shuttle Run) and the vertical jump have a low sensibility to detect functional limitations of the lower extremity.

One of the latest technologies applied to the analysis of muscle properties of the superficial muscles of each individual is Tensyomiography (TMG), which is a diagnostic method that observes the time parameters and the maximum displacement of muscles during contraction.

Its analysis could direct the strength work to be done on bodily structures. The evaluation permits a muscular symmetry or asymmetry to be established, Tc Time (the time that a muscle takes to contract) and Dm (muscular tone or volume), that adopts as lateral and functional symmetry between two muscles or muscle groups above 85%, although in certain muscle groups it can tolerate up to 30% Dm and 15-20% Tc. The implementation of preventive programs directed both at reforcing artromuscular structures as well as the tendinous have proved themselves as extremely efficient.

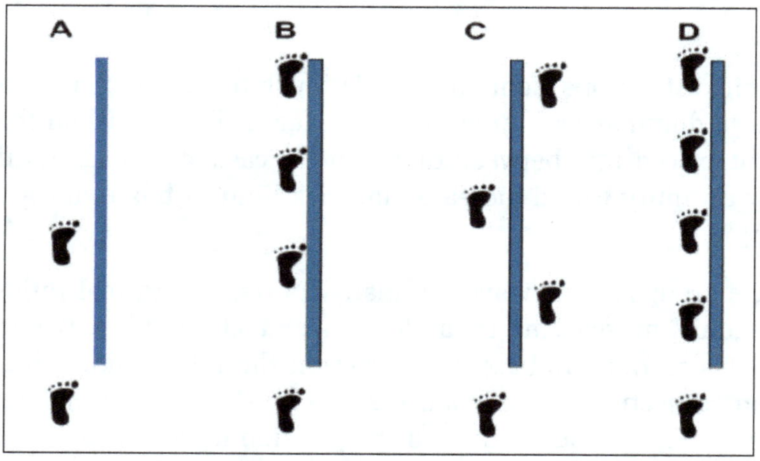

Example of functional tests of one foot jumps in order to evaluate asymmetric functions; A: Single-leg hop for distance, B: Triple hop for distance, C: Crossover triple hop for distance, D: One-legged timed hop.

One of the main biomechanical characteristics of eccentric muscle work is that muscular stretching is obtained whilst producing tension, which implies the stretching of the tendon – muscle, while increasing the levels of muscle strength and improving functional muscle properties at high speed movements. This basis is used in diverse published studies about the prevention of muscle injure in sportspeople, above all, directed at the hamstrings.

Scientific Evidence of the Work Strength as Preventive Work

It is necessary to approach this section distinguishing those experiences centred on the protection of tendon structures and those directed towards muscle function.

Flexibility

The lack of muscle extensibility or the high tone of the antagonist muscle, are factors that enhance sports injuries, especially muscle injure.

Improved Flexibility as Preventive Tool

Muscular injure where no external agent is involved generally occurs during the eccentric phase of muscle contraction. In this case, the muscle develops tension whilst increasing in length. Weakness and fatigue make muscle structures more susceptible to injure when at a specific moment they are incapable of absorbing the generated tension.

When overstretching occurs in a muscle during a quick motor action, its ideal stretching tolerance may be surpassed, jeopardizing its integrity and allowing a possible injury. An imbalance in the level of flexibility in a muscular group, or in the adequate range of movement for the normal actions in the sport, could predispose to injury.

Achieving a correct balance of artromuscular and the structures that make up the locomotor system, as well as achieving an adequately wide level of movements will allow a more fluid movement and coordination in the execution of technical actions and displacements.

Scientific Evidence of the use of Flexibility

The use of flexibility as a prevention method has been a topic of much controversy in the last few years. There are two fundamental strategies that the studies follow to be able to determine the influence of flexibility levels on injuries and, on the other hand, whether improving flexibility could act as an element protective of and preventive from injuries.

Proprioception

A normal joint is dependent on the proper functioning of the neuromuscular control to avoid injury, as this allows dynamic control of the loads applied to it.

General Protocols for Injury Prevention in Sports, Intervention Strategies: Group vs. Individual

The measures successfully introduced in sports to prevent injuries and mentioned previously, allow adequate preventive programs to be designed for each context. This design and its application demand a profound prior reflexion regarding the specific needs of the sportsman/woman with whom the program is to be developed and the best way of tackling the problem.

When introducing a preventive program, one can organise the session or apply the contents of the preventive program in two ways: the first one more generally directed towards dealing with problems generated in each sport, data that will be extracted from the injury profile of the activity and the team sports, being able to organise these programs as parts of the session (warm-up, main part and return to calm) in a group manner. The other direction is more specific and for its organization the individual needs of the sportsperson will be required. It can be done before training with individualised sessions, or reduced group sessions, so as to better attend to their needs.

BASEBALL INJURY PREVENTION

The most common baseball injuries include mild soft tissue injuries, such as muscle pulls (strains), ligament injuries (sprains), cuts, and contusions (bruises). Although baseball is a non-contact sport, most serious injuries are due to contact — either with a ball, bat, or another player.

The repetitive nature of the sport can also cause overuse injuries such as damage to the rotator cuff in the shoulder, or ulnar collateral ligament tears in the elbow.

Proper Preparation for Play

For Coaches

- First aid: Familiarity with first aid, including recognizing and treating the most common injuries, is especially important for coaches. Be able to administer basic first aid for minor injuries, such as facial cuts, bruises, strains, sprains, and tendonitis.
- Field knowledge: Be familiar with your baseball field, including its telephone and cardiac defibrillator.
- Emergency situations: Be prepared for emergencies. Have a plan to reach medical personnel for help with more significant injuries like concussions, breathing problems like wheezing, heat illness, and orthopaedic emergencies, such as fractures and dislocations.
- Follow the rules: Know the rules and encourage safe and appropriate play.

For Players

- Physical exam: A pre-season physical exam is important for both younger and older players. The goal is to prevent injuries and illnesses by identifying any potential medical problems. These may include asthma, allergies, heart, or orthopaedic conditions.
- Warm up: Always take time to warm up. Warm up with some easy calisthenics, such as jumping jacks. Continue with walking or light running, such as running the bases. Many warm-ups also include position-specific stretches. Gentle stretching, in particular your back, hamstrings, and shoulders, can be helpful. Your team coach or athletic trainer may provide a stretching program.
- Cool down and stretch: Stretching at the end of practice is too often neglected because of busy schedules. Stretching can help reduce muscle soreness and keep muscles long and flexible. Slowly and gently stretch after activity, holding each stretch for 30 seconds.

- Hydrate: Even mild levels of dehydration can hurt athletic performance. If you have not had enough fluids, your body will not be able to effectively cool itself through sweat and evaporation. A general recommendation is to drink 24 ounces of non-caffeinated fluid 2 hours before exercise. Drinking an additional 8 ounces of water or sports drink right before exercise is also helpful. While you are exercising, break for an 8 oz. cup of water every 20 minutes.

Ensure Appropriate Equipment and its Use

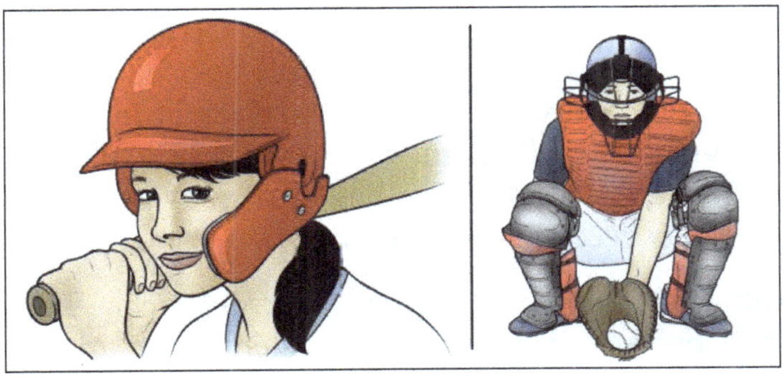

Examples of appropriate safety equipment include a batting helmet with face shield and catcher's protective gear.

- Equipment should fit properly and be worn correctly.
- Wear a batting helmet at the plate, in the "on deck" circle waiting your turn at bat, and during base running.
- Protective face shields attached to batting helmets can reduce the risk of facial injury if hit by a ball.
- Position-specific equipment should be used.
    - Catchers should always use a catcher's mitt, helmet, face mask, throat guard, long-model chest protector, protective supporter, and shin guards.
    - Batters should consider wearing protective jackets to avoid injury from being hit by ball.
- Players should always wear shoes with a snug heel, roomy toe box, good traction, flexibility in the sole, and plenty of ankle support and coverage. Shoes also should breather so as not to encourage bacteria or fungus growth.
- Always break in a new pair of cleats before wearing them during a game, and check shoes periodically for signs of wear and tear. Children often outgrow their shoes before they wear them out.
- Gender-specific equipment may be of value, including athletic supports for boys/men and padded bras for girls/women.

- In youth leagues, softer baseballs decrease the risk of injury from being hit by a pitched ball.
- Players should be instructed in how to avoid getting hit by a ball.

Ensure a Safe Environment

- Inspect the playing field for uneven terrain (holes, divots), glass, and other debris.
- Use a field with breakaway bases. Many injuries occur while sliding into bases. The traditional stationary base is a rigid obstacle for an athlete to encounter while sliding. In contrast, a breakaway base is snapped onto grommets attached to an anchored rubber mat, which holds it in place during normal play. Although a sliding runner can dislodge it, the breakaway base is stable and will not detach during normal base running. Installing breakaway bases on all playing fields could significantly decrease sliding injuries.
- Assess weather conditions and be prepared to delay/cancel the game, especially in cases of particularly hot weather or thunderstorms with lightning.

Focus on Technique

Base Running

The American Academy of Orthopaedic Surgeons recommends the following tips for those individuals sliding into, as well as protecting, the bases while playing baseball and softball:

- Players under age 10 should not be taught to slide.
- Proper instruction in sliding technique must be provided and players must practice sliding, beginning with a sliding bag, before being allowed to slide during a game.
- The "obstruction" rule (the fielding player cannot obstruct the path of the runner) must be taught and observed. Getting in the way of the runner or blocking the base without possession of the ball is dangerous to both the runner and fielder.
- To prevent foot and ankle injuries between the runner and fielder on first base, a "double bag" (a separate bag for each team one white, one orange) should be used so both the runner and first baseman have their own base.

Pitching and Throwing

Follow established guidelines for youth baseball, which include limiting the number of pitches thrown and type of pitches thrown, according to age.

Both coaches and parents should be responsive to young pitchers who complain of arm or shoulder pain. Be sure to seek out medical care for arm pain that does not go away or that comes back every time a child resumes pitching.

Prevent Overuse Injuries

Because many young athletes are focusing on just one sport and are training year-round, doctors are seeing an increase in overuse injuries. The American Academy of Orthopaedic Surgeons has partnered with STOP Sports Injuries to help educate parents, coaches, and athletes about how to prevent overuse injuries. Specific tips to prevent overuse injuries in baseball include:

- Limit the number of teams in which your child is playing in one season. Kids who play on more than one team are especially at risk for overuse injuries.
- Do not allow your child to play one sport year round — taking regular breaks and playing other sports is essential to skill development and injury prevention.
- Do not allow your child to pitch on consecutive days and avoid pitching on multiple teams with overlapping seasons.

Injury Diagnosis

Good communication between doctors, players, parents, and coaches is key to diagnosing and treating more significant baseball injuries.

Young players may not be able to recall exactly how an injury happened or describe their symptoms in detail. They may even hide injuries because of concern about being removed from play.

Coaches and parents must pay close attention to changes in a player's participation or performance. Should there be an injury, doctors may need their help to provide accurate details and a medical history.

Safe Return to Play

An injured player's symptoms must be completely gone before returning to play. For example:

- In case of a joint problem, the player must have no pain, no swelling, full range of motion, and normal strength.
- In case of concussion, the player must have no symptoms at rest or with exercise, and should be cleared by the appropriate medical provider.
- In case of a shoulder or elbow overuse injury, the player should gradually return to a throwing program, increasing the number of throws depending on the length of time away from play, and their specific team position.

INJURY PREVENTION IN FOOTBALL

Injury prevention seemed to be an area consisting of multiple topics.

We believe that working in each of the following areas will (of course) not account for injuries after contact/foul, however, might prevent from non-contact injuries.

Screening for Injury History

Player with an injuries in the past player are more likely to injure themselves again at the same site.

Therefore injury history can give insight into player's likelihood of re-injury (and body site) and strength and conditioners can target specific muscles that have been shown problematic in the past and/or to stabilize specific joints, such as the ankle.

Strength Training

Besides strength training for enhancing performance, it can also have emphasis on injury prevention. It seems that eccentric muscle contractions showed high muscle activation, put high stress on the muscle, and therefore also seemed to have the highest preventive effect.

Eccentric hamstring exercises were reported effective in preventing hamstring strains and fatigue.

A second goal in strength training with an injury prevention emphasis is to work on a) muscle and b) leg asymmetries.

- Hamstring to Quadriceps strength asymmetries (measured as eccentric hamstring to concentric quadriceps ratio or concentric hamstring versus concentric quadriceps) were shown to significantly impact injury incidence.

  A Hamstring to quadriceps ratio of below 0.75 - 0.6 seemed to be "problematic" and suggested a higher probability of future injury. Also, the speed of movement/testing seemed crucial. Higher velocities seemed to be more prone to show higher ratios.

  However, considering the true speed of movement during kicking/football testing at higher velocities seemed to make sense. Additionally, preferred versus non-preferred legs should be investigated.

  Information in youth players in both genders are also present throughout the literature, suggesting greater development for quadriceps muscle compared to hamstring for girls after menarche and therefore a higher risk for ACL injury.

As a result, hamstring strengthening should be instituted for girls after menarche.

- Dominant to non-dominant leg muscle strength (10-12) differences but also anatomical/functional leg length differences seemed to impact injury incidence.

  Interestingly, experienced players with longer professional training age showed a more balanced use of their lower extremities to cope with previously developed musculoskeletal asymmetries and possibly reduce injury risk.

Warm-up

The general purpose of the warm-up is to increase blood circulation to the working muscle to meet the increased oxygen demand. As a result, the activity will result in increasing tissue temperature, which helps electrical and chemical reactions in the muscle. Decreased resistance of muscle and joints, increased thermoregulatory strain, faster nerve conduction rate, improved rate of muscle contraction and reaction time, altered force-velocity relationship, increased anaerobic energy provision increases with temperature as well.

Generally, three different types of warm-up exists:

- Passive warm-up such as hot showers or heat from the environment (heat pads, sun). This type of warm-up is not necessarily recommended as it increases the blood flow to the skin instead of to the muscle. However, physical activity in heat will have an effect on performance.
- General warm-up consists of jogging, cycling and every other activity in which the major muscle groups are involved. General warm-ups have been proven to have greater impact on short term performance and intermediate (>10 seconds, but <5 minutes) and long term (>5 minutes), if the actual activity is started in a non-fatigue state and if thermoregulatory procedures are still limited.

Specific Warm-up

With regard to a football specific background, specific warm-up consists of different movements with and without the ball that are typical in football. Advantages of specific warm-up are an integration of skills and its neural activation/responses.

The effect of warm-up procedures on injury rate were seen in female youth football players. The warm-up consisted of the F-Marc programm from FIFA or basic components in stretching, strengthening, plyometrics, and change of direction.

Teams with a higher compliance to the programm showed a 35% lower risk of injury as well as coaches who incorporated injury prevention programs presented a 46% decrease in injury risk.

Interestingly, muscle temperature following a warm-up has been shown to last up to 45 minutes.

Cooling down/Recovery

A variety of cool-downs/recovery procedures exist. The available time and purpose will decide over the recovery procedure.

Monitoring Players

Monitoring players can have various forms, but the purpose is more or less the same - to control the prescribed stimulus and avoid overtraining, overuse, and finally chronic fatigue.

The problem in monitoring players is that exercise/training prescription is often based on external factors (duration of exercise, repetitions and frequencies) that are external (factors that are opposed onto athletes) and the internal load for each player various tremendously for the same exercise. Therefore it is necessary to quantify the internal load.

As a result training load of players can be monitoring through a) external and/or b) internal load.

External Load

The easiest and simple choice to monitor players is to record the duration and type of activity during training.

Furthermore, accumulation of training hours might have implications in a long-term-player-development and therefore should be monitored throughout the players' development.

Depending on the environment, if football circuits and/or interval training is used, the training load can be measured via distances covered, number of runs, average velocities etc. As a result and in that particular situation the load is known as well and can be altered easily. This approach is very practical during pre-season to systematically increase load.

The "latest" technology whilst monitoring players is GPS units (or any other time-motion-analysis technology). The devices are able to track players, measure distances, accelerations and decelerations (and total body load). GPS units are also available in real-time modus, can be synchronized with heart rate monitors and therefore, both build a good combination to assess external (GPS) + internal (hear rate) load. However, the reliability for high intensity running and very high intensity running was poor.

Still, training prescription can be based on time-motion-analysis if time and manpower are available to handle the data. GPS units (and heart rate systems) are quite expensive and therefore not suited for all environments.

Internal Load

Heart rate as a measure of internal load is well established. Durations in different heart rate zones (usually expressed as % of max heart rate) will determine the load and training can be implemented accordingly. If real time monitoring is presented, session can be stopped when certain duration in certain heart rate zone is fulfilled.

Ratio of perceived exertion (RPE), as a subjective method to measure internal load was originally developed by Borg et al. and further developed as the so-called session-RPE.

The session-RPE is calculated by multiplying the RPE of the session with its duration and was proven to correlate with heart rate, VO2 and accumulation of blood lactate and was used in a football setting.

Measuring hormonal and immunological (cortisol, testosterone, noradrenaline, IgA, IgG, IgM), reactions were also measured in a football setting.

Another form of monitoring (psychological) stress was to evaluate sleep, mood, mistrust, trait anxiety, coping and the significant predictors/variables could explain 23% of injuries occurrence.

Typical content for an injury prevention program was:

- Jogging, skippings, running backwards and carioca.
- Stretching, hamstrings, quadriceps, inner thighs and hip flexor.
- Strengthening of the same muscles.
- Plyometrics, variations of hopping jumping and bounding.
- Agility/Change of direction.

Generally, we feel that the described exercise can be put into a more football specific context, involving the ball and the program can easily be implemented into the warm-up.

SOCCER INJURY PREVENTION

Already the most popular international team sport, soccer continues to gain popularity in the United States. With more people playing soccer, it is not surprising that the number of soccer-related injuries is increasing — particularly as children get older and their level of play intensifies.

Sprains and strains, often around the knee and ankle, are very common in soccer. Player collisions — either full body or kick collisions — can cause a wide range of injuries, including cuts, bruises, and concussions. Overuse injuries, such as Achilles tendinitis and shin splints, frequently occur, as well.

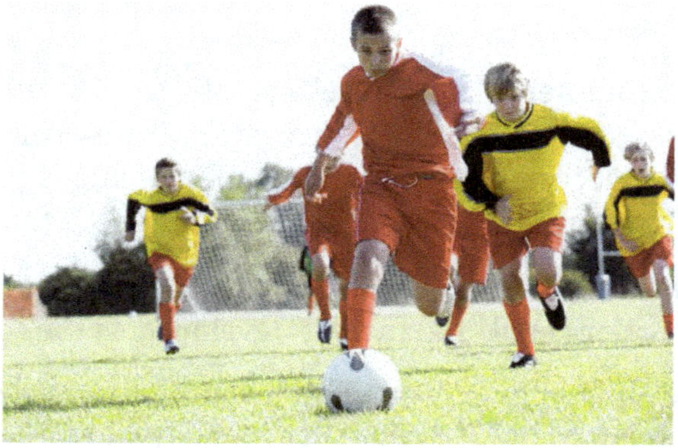

Several strategies can help prevent soccer injuries — from careful inspection of the field to wearing proper shin guards.

Proper Preparation for Play

- Maintain fitness: Be sure you are in good physical condition at the start of soccer season. During the off-season, stick to a balanced fitness program that incorporates aerobic exercise, strength training, and flexibility. If you are out of shape at the start of the season, gradually increase your activity level and slowly build back up to a higher fitness level.
- Warm up: Always take time to warm up. Research studies show that cold muscles are more prone to injury. Warm up with jumping jacks, or running or walking in place for 3 to 5 minutes. Many warm-ups also include sport- or position-specific stretches. If your warm-up includes stretching, be sure to perform them slowly and gently, holding each stretch for 30 seconds. Ballistic, "bouncing" stretches are usually not recommended.
- Cool down and stretch: Stretching at the end of practice is too often neglected because of busy schedules. Stretching can help reduce muscle soreness and keep muscles long and flexible. Be sure to stretch after each training practice to reduce your risk for injury.
- Hydrate: Even mild levels of dehydration can hurt athletic performance. If you have not had enough fluids, your body will not be able to effectively cool itself through sweat and evaporation. A general recommendation is to drink 24 ounces of non-caffeinated fluid 2 hours before exercise. Drinking an additional 8 ounces of water or sports drink right before exercise is also helpful. While you are exercising, break for an 8 oz. cup of water every 20 minutes.

Ensure Appropriate Equipment

- Wear shin guards to help protect your lower legs. Soccer tournament records show that lower leg injuries are most often caused by inadequate shin guards.

- Wear shoes with molded cleats or ribbed soles. Shoes with screw-in cleats often are associated with a higher risk of injury. However, shoes with screw-in cleats should be worn when more traction is needed, such as on a wet field with high grass.
- Use synthetic, nonabsorbent balls on wet playing fields. Leather balls can become water-logged and very heavy when wet, putting players at high risk for injury.

Ensure a Safe Environment

- Soccer goals should be well padded and properly secured: Padding the goal decreases the incidence of head injuries when the goalie and other team members collide with the posts.
- The playing surface must be kept in good condition: Holes on the playing field should be filled, bare spots reseeded, and debris removed.
- Secure the goals at the end of play: A simple bicycle lock can chain the goals together and prevent them from tipping over. Unsecured, unsupervised soccer goals can fall onto children and result in severe injuries.
- Pay attention to the weather conditions: In a thunderstorm, leave the field and get inside immediately. In hot weather, take sufficient water breaks. In cold weather, wear appropriate clothing, including gloves and hats. Consider shortening practices in severe temperature extremes.
- Do not crawl under or sit on the goal, or hang from the net: Injuries and deaths have occurred when goals have fallen onto players.

Prepare for Injuries

- Coaches should be knowledgeable about first aid and be able to administer it for minor injuries, such as facial cuts, bruises, or minor strains and sprains.
- If playing on artificial grass fields, make sure to adequately clean any skin scrapes or abrasions to reduce the chance of them getting infected.
- Be prepared for emergencies. All coaches should have a plan to reach medical personnel for help with more significant injuries such as concussions, dislocations, contusions, sprains, abrasions, and fractures.

Safe Return to Play

An injured player's symptoms must be completely gone before returning to play. For example:

- In case of a joint problem, the player must have no pain, no swelling, full range of motion, and normal strength.

- In case of concussion, the player must have no symptoms at rest or with exercise, and should be cleared by the appropriate medical provider.

Prevent Overuse Injuries

Because many young athletes are focusing on just one sport and are training year-round, doctors are seeing an increase in overuse injuries. The American Academy of Orthopaedic Surgeons has partnered with STOP Sports Injuries to help educate parents, coaches, and athletes about how to prevent overuse injuries. Specific tips to prevent overuse injuries include:

- Limit the number of teams in which your child is playing in one season. Kids who play on more than one team are especially at risk for overuse injuries.
- Do not allow your child to play one sport year round — taking regular breaks and playing other sports is essential to skill development and injury prevention.

PREVENTION OF CLIMBING INJURIES

Have a Daily Prevention Program

Perform Static Stretches

Due to the repetitive nature of climbing, your muscles can become overdeveloped and tight. Tight muscles can pull and strain the tendons where they attach to the bone, and can increase resistance to movement. This makes it more challenging to reach distant holds with your arms and legs. Static stretching on a daily basis is an effective way to lengthen your muscles and increase your overall flexibility. Static stretches are typically held for up to 30 seconds. Make sure to stretch your hips, shoulders, wrists and fingers.

Perform Antagonist Exercises

Antagonist muscles oppose the muscles that you primarily use to climb. They create movement in the opposite direction. Weak antagonist muscles can leave you highly susceptible to overuse injury. Strengthening your antagonist muscles daily balances your body and can decrease the likelihood of getting hurt. Exercises such as rowing, triceps presses, and wrist and finger extensions help develop your antagonist muscles.

Warm up Properly

Dynamic Stretches before Climbing

Dynamic stretching is the most effective method of stretching prior to an activity. The stretch is performed by taking the muscle through a full range of motion lasting 2-3 seconds and then returning to the starting position. It is important to perform dynamic stretching for ten minutes prior to climbing on the wall. Dynamic stretching will increase the blood flow to your muscles, tendons and joints, and can help prevent injury.

Train Like you Climb

Engage in Mirror Movement

Many training exercises don't reflect your body's position while climbing and therefore don't translate into meaningful climbing improvements. In order for an exercise to carry over to climbing, the body position in the exercise must be similar to the body position when you climb. Exercising in this way will produce more meaningful results.

Be Mindful of your Movement

Learn Correct Climbing Technique

- Keep good posture,
- Bring your hips into the wall,
- Straighten your arms,
- Push with your feet,
- Climb like you crawl.

Listen to your Body

Allow Adequate Recovery Tim

If an area of your body is sore or feels tweaked, rest and allow it to recover. Although recovery time is highly variable for each individual, many climbers need at least 48 hours to fully recover from a challenging workout. If you are feeling overly fatigued after training sessions and have some minor pain, don't just climb through it. Take the time to rest and rehabilitate so that you can continue to climb injury free.

PERMISSIONS

All chapters in this book are published with permission under the Creative Commons Attribution Share Alike License or equivalent. Every chapter published in this book has been scrutinized by our experts. Their significance has been extensively debated. The topics covered herein carry significant information for a comprehensive understanding. They may even be implemented as practical applications or may be referred to as a beginning point for further studies.

We would like to thank the editorial team for lending their expertise to make the book truly unique. They have played a crucial role in the development of this book. Without their invaluable contributions this book wouldn't have been possible. They have made vital efforts to compile up to date information on the varied aspects of this subject to make this book a valuable addition to the collection of many professionals and students.

This book was conceptualized with the vision of imparting up-to-date and integrated information in this field. To ensure the same, a matchless editorial board was set up. Every individual on the board went through rigorous rounds of assessment to prove their worth. After which they invested a large part of their time researching and compiling the most relevant data for our readers.

The editorial board has been involved in producing this book since its inception. They have spent rigorous hours researching and exploring the diverse topics which have resulted in the successful publishing of this book. They have passed on their knowledge of decades through this book. To expedite this challenging task, the publisher supported the team at every step. A small team of assistant editors was also appointed to further simplify the editing procedure and attain best results for the readers.

Apart from the editorial board, the designing team has also invested a significant amount of their time in understanding the subject and creating the most relevant covers. They scrutinized every image to scout for the most suitable representation of the subject and create an appropriate cover for the book.

The publishing team has been an ardent support to the editorial, designing and production team. Their endless efforts to recruit the best for this project, has resulted in the accomplishment of this book. They are a veteran in the field of academics and their pool of knowledge is as vast as their experience in printing. Their expertise and guidance has proved useful at every step. Their uncompromising quality standards have made this book an exceptional effort. Their encouragement from time to time has been an inspiration for everyone.

The publisher and the editorial board hope that this book will prove to be a valuable piece of knowledge for students, practitioners and scholars across the globe.

INDEX

A

Achilles Tendinopathy, 31, 97
Adenosine Triphosphate, 132, 142
Amenorrhea, 78, 82-83, 85
Amino Acids, 129, 131, 133-134, 138-142, 146-151, 154-155
Ammonia Buffering, 131, 134
Androstenedione, 129
Ankle Taping, 38, 41-42
Anterior Cruciate Ligament, 29, 65, 72, 90, 97, 203
Arginine, 139-141, 147
Arterial Gas Embolism, 17, 20-21, 23
Arthritis, 11, 30, 66, 68, 161-162
Athletic Heart Syndrome, 36, 75-76

B

Bankart Lesion, 34
Biceps Tendinitis, 109
Bursa Inflammation, 68-69

C

Calcaneofibular, 32, 36-37
Carbohydrate Content, 121-122, 124-125, 128, 155
Cardiopulmonary Physical Therapy, 164
Chiropractic Care, 12
Cold Therapy, 40, 46
Compression Wrap, 40, 46
Conconi Test, 16
Creatine, 65, 130, 134, 140-146, 148

D

Decompression Sickness, 17, 20-23
Deltoid Ligament, 36, 44
Diving Medicine, 1, 17-19, 22-26
Dopamine, 131, 133

E

Electrolyte Balance, 124-125
Ephedra, 129-130
Ergogenic Aids, 129, 145
Extracorporeal Shock Waves Therapy, 31

F

Femoroacetabular Impingement, 30
Finger Pulley Tears, 112-113
Fluid Balance, 122, 125, 156, 158

G

Geriatric Physical Therapy, 163
Glutamine, 131-142, 150
Gluteal Muscles, 88, 99, 106
Glycaemic Index, 121
Groin Strain, 36, 44, 46-47, 96

H

Heart Rate Monitor, 17
Hyperbaric Oxygen Therapy, 18, 22-23, 25
Hypertonic Drink, 160

I

Ibuprofen, 46, 50, 67, 69, 77, 105
Isokinetic Test, 63-64
Isoleucine, 139-141
Isotonic Drinks, 157-160

K

Knee Flexion, 53-54, 65
Krebs Cycle, 132, 134, 136

L

Ligament Sprains, 37, 169
Losartan, 62

M

Magnetic Resonance Imaging, 50-51, 56, 151
Munich Classification, 58-59
Muscular Endurance, 2, 141, 144, 176-177
Musculoskeletal System, 10, 28, 167

N

Naproxen, 50, 67, 69
Nitrogen Narcosis, 19-21

O

Orthopedic Surgery, 6, 8, 29

Osteoporosis, 3, 11, 68, 78, 80-81, 83, 85-86, 162
Oxidative Stress, 131, 133-135, 138

P
Patellofemoral Pain Syndrome, 87, 89-90, 99
Pediatric Physical Therapy, 163
Plantar Fasciitis, 103-104
Plasma Glutamine, 131, 133, 136, 139
Posterior Cruciate Ligament, 30, 65, 97
Pulmonary Barotrauma, 20-21

R
Rectus Abdominus, 179

S
Serotonin, 131, 133-134, 139-140
Shin Pain, 36, 48-50
Shoulder Subluxation, 92, 113
Soy Protein, 148-149, 151
Sport Psychology, 1, 13-14, 35
Sports Chiropractor, 12
Sports Hernia, 178
Sports Hypnosis, 15
Sports Physiotherapy, 1, 8-9
Sports Supplements, 129, 131
Stress Fracture, 2, 49-51, 86, 107

T
Therapeutic Exercises, 9, 161, 164, 174-176
Thermotherapy, 169
Tryptophan, 133, 139-140

U
Undersea And Hyperbaric Medicine, 17, 24, 26

V
Valine, 139-141
Vestibular Rehabilitation, 163